MULTIPLE SCLEROSIS

**Recent Titles in the
Biographies of Disease Series**

ADHD
Paul Graves Hammerness

Anorexia
Stacy Beller Stryer

Autism
Lisa D. Benaron

Cancer
Susan E. Pories, Marsha A. Moses, and Margaret M. Lotz

Fibromyalgia
Kim D. Jones and Janice H. Hoffman

Influenza
Roni K. Devlin

Obesisty
Kathleen Y. Wolin, Sc.D., and Jennifer M. Petrelli

Polio
Daniel J. Wilson

Rabies
P. Dileep Kumar

Sports Injuries
Jennifer A. Baima

MULTIPLE SCLEROSIS

Lisa I. Iezzoni

Biographies of Disease
Julie K. Silver, M.D., Series Editor

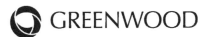
GREENWOOD

AN IMPRINT OF ABC-CLIO, LLC
Santa Barbara, California • Denver, Colorado • Oxford, England

Library of Congress Cataloging-in-Publication Data

Iezzoni, Lisa I.
    Multiple sclerosis / Lisa I. Iezzoni.
        p. ; cm. — (Biographies of disease)
    Includes bibliographical references and index.
    ISBN 978-0-313-36564-5 (hard copy : alk. paper) — ISBN 978-0-313-36565-2
    (EISBN)
1. Multiple sclerosis. I. Title. II. Series: Biographies of disease.
[DNLM: 1. Multiple Sclerosis. WL 360 I22m 2010]
RC377.I29   2010
616.8′00—dc22   2009050710

ISBN: 978-0-313-36564-5
EISBN: 978-0-313-36565-2

14 13 12 11 10   1 2 3 4 5

This book is also available on the World Wide Web as an eBook.
Visit www.abc-clio.com for details.

Greenwood
An Imprint of ABC-CLIO, LLC

ABC-CLIO, LLC
130 Cremona Drive, P.O. Box 1911
Santa Barbara, California 93116-1911

This book is printed on acid-free paper ∞

Manufactured in the United States of America

Contents

Series Foreword

E very disease has a story to tell: about how it started long ago and began to disable or even take the lives of its innocent victims, about the way it hurts us, and about how we are trying to stop it. In this Biographies of Disease series, the authors tell the stories of the diseases that we have come to know and dread.

The stories of these diseases have all of the components that make for great literature. There is incredible drama played out in real-life scenes from the past, present, and future. You'll read about how men and women of science stumbled trying to save the lives of those they aimed to protect. Turn the pages and you'll also learn about the amazing success of those who fought for health and won, often saving thousands of lives in the process.

If you don't want to be a health professional or research scientist now, when you finish this book you may think differently. The men and women in this book are heroes who often risked their own lives to save or improve ours. This is the biography of a disease, but it is also the story of real people who made incredible sacrifices to stop it in its tracks.

Julie K. Silver, M.D.
Assistant Professor, Harvard Medical School
Department of Physical Medicine and Rehabilitation

Preface

"MS, crippler of young adults."

That phrase kept circling my mind during the winter break after my first semester at Harvard Medical School in December 1980. After four years of off-and-on symptoms—strange, shadowy sensations that would appear suddenly, last for a few weeks or months, and then vanish, only to recur again months later—I had finally gone to a neurologist, a doctor specializing in the nervous system (the brain, spinal cord, and nerves that control bodily functions). For those four years, I had dismissed these weird episodes, attributing the odd sensations to stress. After all, I had been taking intensive pre-med and other graduate courses, as well as working to pay for my housing and food, and I was much too busy to think about anything else. I was in my early twenties and had always been strong and healthy. The notion of having some disease never crossed my mind.

In addition, the fleeting symptoms were so strange, hard to describe and understand. Who would believe my story? During July 1978 when I was taking summer school chemistry, for example, two symptoms arrived simultaneously. While I was jogging along the Charles River, which winds between Boston and Cambridge, Massachusetts, I didn't know where my legs were in space. Of course my legs were where they had always been—pumping along, carrying my body over my several-mile running route. But unless I looked down and saw them, I didn't know their position. Furthermore, my legs felt as if someone had taken a red-hot branding iron and pressed it into my flesh—a painful sensation of searing heat. My skin was not particularly red or warm to the touch, but the sensations seemed real nonetheless. Weeks later, these feelings disappeared, only to return months afterward. This cycle repeated itself several times over the next few years.

Within weeks after starting medical school, the symptoms came back with a vengeance and a twist impossible to ignore. My internal gyroscope—unconscious processes that kept me balanced, upright, and moving forward—felt off. While walking along, I would veer involuntarily into stationary objects, such as trees or parked cars. A stranger watching me might think I was drunk, unable to control my movements. Something was clearly wrong, and I decided to consult a neurologist.

On that December day, the neurologist at the University Health Services was gentle, kind, and cautious, and he took me very seriously. He listened carefully as I recounted several years of odd symptoms that would come and go. He said I would need to undergo several diagnostic tests to make sure I did not have a brain tumor or some other disease. However, he had a strong suspicion about my diagnosis. My story, he said, fit the classic history of multiple sclerosis, MS, but he wouldn't know for certain until all the tests were done.

So I went on my winter break with those letters and the fund-raising slogan of the day—used by charitable organizations to solicit donations for MS research and advocacy—revolving in my mind. "MS, crippler of young adults." What was MS? What did this diagnosis mean for me?

* * * * *

Multiple sclerosis (MS) is a degenerative disease of the central nervous system, and it has no cure. Its origins in the powerful and mysterious central nervous system—the brain and spinal cord, which dictate and regulate wide-ranging bodily functions—account for the profound, diverse, and hard-to-describe symptoms I had experienced. The words "multiple sclerosis" suggest, quite literally, how the disease damages critical brain and spinal cord tissues:

- "Multiple" indicates the disease affects more than one area of the brain and/or spinal cord; and
- "Sclerosis" means hardening, which describes changes or plaques in the myelin sheath, the protective protein sleeve or outer layer that insulates nerves in the brain and spinal cord.

Beyond this basic understanding, however, much about MS remains a mystery, just like the central nervous system where it resides. Although many theories speculate about what causes MS, no one yet knows for certain why the disease affects one person versus another. No one has found a way to stop the plaques from forming or to reverse the damage and cure the disease. Most importantly for someone like me in December 1980, no one can tell most individual patients newly diagnosed with MS exactly how the disease will affect their health and daily lives. The manifestations of MS over a lifetime vary widely. At one extreme, some people experience mild or moderate periodic symptoms for many years. At the other extreme, the disease causes paralysis, debility, and rarely even death. Most persons, though, have a fairly normal life expectancy. Thus, to live with MS is to live with uncertainty, possibly for many decades.

MS is relatively rare compared with many other diseases. It affects between 250,000 and 350,000 persons in the United States, which has a population of about 300 million people: approximately 1 person in 1,000 has MS. As indicated by the fund-raising slogan, MS is most often diagnosed in young or middle-aged adults. MS thus arrives just as people are finishing school, starting careers, building intimate relationships, and beginning families.

Given this timing and the disability frequently caused by MS, the effects of the disease often ripple outward, like concentric waves of water after a pebble is tossed into a pond. At the center is the person with MS, but his or her spouse or partner, children, parents, other family members, friends, and neighbors can become involved and feel the consequences of this disabling disease. Thus, MS touches many more people than the several hundred thousand individuals with the condition. Treatments may ease certain symptoms of MS and perhaps slow progression of the disease. But the way that these social networks and communities respond, such as by making public transportation, shops, and other buildings accessible and welcoming to individuals with disabilities, also have important implications for the quality of life of persons living for decades with MS.

As a volume in the *Biography of Disease* series, this book offers an introduction to MS. Chapter 1 describes where MS strikes in the body: the central nervous system, with its complex conscious and unconscious functions. Chapter 2 provides a history of how MS was discovered and how ideas about it have changed over time and are still evolving today. Chapter 3 presents the epidemiology of MS: the characteristics of persons getting the disease and locations around the world with especially high rates of illness. Chapter 4 discusses the potential role of the immune system in causing MS. Chapter 5 describes symptoms of MS and how the disease is diagnosed. Chapter 6 introduces treatments for MS, including both medications and complementary and alternative therapy. Chapter 7 reviews rehabilitation therapies, while Chapter 8 discusses the role of mobility aids, such as walkers and different types of wheelchairs. Chapter 9 concludes the book by discussing broader societal issues relating to disability civil rights and environmental factors that allow persons, even with significant disabilities, to live safely and productively in their homes and communities. A timeline of critical discoveries and events relating to MS is presented. A glossary, which defines scientific terms used throughout this book, appears at the back; a list of common acronyms appears in the front. A list of relevant Internet Web sites and a bibliography of selected books and articles used in preparing this book are also included. To clarify key facts or concepts, pictures appear throughout the book drawn by Anil Shukla, MD, a young emergency room doctor who moon-lights as a medical illustrator.

In this book, I tell stories of men and women with MS whom I have inter-viewed for research projects (Iezzoni, 2003; Iezzoni and O'Day, 2006). To protect their privacy, I do not use their real names but instead call them by pseudonyms (made-up names). As in this preface, I also occasionally recount my own experi-ences. These personal stories show how MS affects actual people and give their perspectives on the disease and related disability. Nevertheless, it is important to remember that—as emphasized above—MS is a very variable disease. Differ-ent people have different experiences with MS.

This book introduces a complex and mysterious disease. Much about MS remains unknown, and there is no cure. The uncertainty of MS is omnipresent for persons with the disease, something they deal with every day. For scientists, researchers, and doctors, these mysteries and uncertainties pose fascinating chal-lenges. Future discoveries may someday prevent MS and improve the lives of per-sons living with this frequently debilitating disease.

List of Illustrations

List of Tables

Acronyms

ACTH	adrenocorticotropic hormone
ADA	Americans with Disabilities Act
CFR	Code of Federal Regulations
CIL	center for independent living
CSF	cerebrospinal fluid
CT	computerized tomography
DME	durable medical equipment
EBV	Epstein-Barr virus
EDSS	Expanded Disability Status Scale
FDA	Food and Drug Administration
HLA	human leukocyte antigen
MHC	major histocompatibility complex
MRI	magnetic resonance imaging
MS	multiple sclerosis
NIAID	National Institute of Allergy and Infectious Diseases
NINDS	National Institute of Neurological Diseases and Stroke
NMSS	National Multiple Sclerosis Society
PML	progressive mutifocal leukoencephalopathy

1

Introducing the Central Nervous System and the Pathology of Multiple Sclerosis

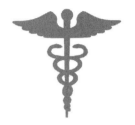

Multiple sclerosis (MS) is a degenerative disease of the central nervous system. Here, the adjective degenerative means progressive deterioration of specialized cells, tissues, or organ systems such that they no longer function normally. When the central nervous system becomes impaired, no longer functioning as it normally does, persons can experience countless different symptoms, physical difficulties, and cognitive problems. Therefore, learning about MS must start with a basic understanding of the central nervous system.

Chapter 1 begins by describing the gross anatomy (major structures visible to the human eye) of the central nervous system. Because of the distinctive appearance of these soft tissues, scientists have described the central nervous system as made of white matter and gray matter. The chapter then looks at the histology (microscopic anatomy) of nerve cells and their neighboring supportive cells, which allow the central nervous system to perform its essential functions. Differing aspects of millions of cells combine to give specific components of the central nervous system their characteristic white and gray appearance. The damaging degenerative processes (pathology) that cause MS involve nerve cells, other related cells, and their microscopic surrounding structures within the central nervous system. Although each individual damaged cell structure is microscopic, when disease affects many cells, the destruction becomes obvious to the human eye. MS is often called a "white matter disease," and this chapter explains why.

Before beginning, one caveat is necessary. Neuroanatomy and neurohistology (neuro indicates relating to the nervous system) are incredibly complex (Kiernan, 2009). Scientists have written entire books simply about the gross anatomy and histology of the brain and spinal cord. This chapter provides only the briefest overview. The human brain and spinal cord each have specific regions and structures that perform very particular tasks, such as maintaining proper internal organ functioning; receiving and formulating sensory information involving vision, hearing, touch, and smell; forming and processing conscious thoughts; reasoning to contemplate complex problems; producing intelligible and meaningful speech; experiencing and reacting to different types of emotions; stabilizing the body and being aware of the body's position in space; feeling pain; and intentionally moving specific muscles. Through decades of careful study, neurologists and neuroscientists have mapped these innumerable tasks and functions to specific locations in the brain and spinal cord—an effort that continues today.

Mastering this anatomic and functional complexity allows skilled neurologists to pinpoint where lesions might exist in a patient's nervous system. Based only on a patient's description of the bodily location and nature of his or her symptoms, followed by a thorough physical examination, an expert neurologist can speculate with some certainty about where abnormalities have occurred in the brain or spinal cord. Before radiographic tests, such as computerized tomography (CT) scans or magnetic resonance imaging (MRI), became available, with their clear anatomical images of neurological structures, neurologists relied only on their detailed understanding of neuroanatomy to localize disease (see Chapter 2). Neurology thus developed a reputation of being a highly intellectual and deductive field along the lines of rigorous detective work—knowing the terrain and linking together disparate clues to deduce if and where a crime (in this case, a disease) has happened. Superb anatomical knowledge, keen observational abilities, and superior physical examination skills make the best diagnostic detectives.

OVERVIEW OF THE NERVOUS SYSTEM

The nervous system is the circuitry of the body, with millions of infinitesimal filaments reaching virtually all structures, from visible organs to microscopic tissues. It both sends and receives electrical and chemical messages to control unconscious organ functioning and carry out conscious, intentional actions. The nervous system has two broad components: the central nervous system and the peripheral nervous system. As described below, the central nervous system is the brain and the spinal cord. Because of its special role, the central nervous system is carefully protected by anatomic structures and cushioned by constantly circulating fluid. The peripheral nervous system encompasses the myriad nerves outside the brain and spinal cord that carry out the instructions coming from that central overseer. Nerve cells from the central nervous system send chemical or electrical signals to their peripheral nervous system partners, telling them what to do.

The specific cells that make up the peripheral nervous system are similar to those in the central nervous system. However, some important differences do exist, highlighting the complexity of the nervous system and its operations. In addition, the different cell types interact in somewhat different ways in the central versus peripheral nervous systems. Certain disorders, such as diabetes mellitus, herpes zoster (shingles), myasthenia gravis, and complications from certain drugs (including ethanol poisoning), involve the peripheral nervous system. Because MS is a disease of the central nervous system, this chapter focuses there.

CENTRAL NERVOUS SYSTEM ANATOMY

In vertebrate animals, the central nervous system consists of the brain and the spinal cord, which are continuous structures (see Figure 1.1). As its name suggests, the central nervous system functions as the body's central command unit. It receives information from inside and outside the body and transmits messages outward to control body functions—both conscious (such as muscle movements to perform voluntary, intentional actions) and unconscious (such as controlling heart and lung functions). The brain is also the seat of thought, learning, memory, emotion, reasoning, and numerous other mental processes. A large and complex brain distinguishes human beings from all other creatures.

Given their critical roles, the soft, gelatinous brain and spinal cord are protected by bony structures. The skull, with its smooth thick vault of bone, encases the brain. The spinal cord is continuous with the medulla section of the brain, exiting the skull through the foramen magnum, a large opening at the base of the skull.

The bones protecting the spinal cord—a long cylindrical structure with 31 pairs of spinal nerves—are more complicated. The spinal cord passes downward along the vertebral canal, a passageway through openings in the vertebrae, the bones that make up the backbone or spine. Starting from the top, the human spine has 7 vertebrae in the cervical or neck region, 12 vertebrae in the thoracic or chest area, 5 vertebrae in the lumbar or lower back area, and 5 vertebrae fused together making up the sacrum (sacral region). The spine terminates in a small bone called the coccyx.

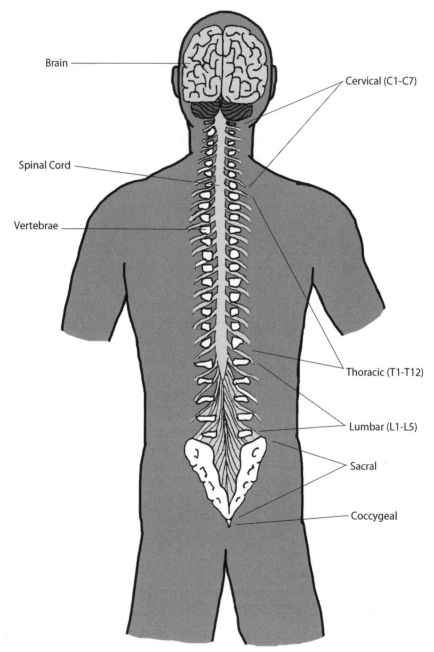

Brain

Cervical (C1-C7)

Spinal Cord

Vertebrae

Thoracic (T1-T12)

Lumbar (L1-L5)

Sacral

Coccygeal

Figure 1.1. Central Nervous System. The brain and spinal cord comprise the central nervous system. The spinal cord passes downward through the vertebral canal, with 31 pairs of spinal nerves emerging on either side to send and receive messages between the brain and the body. [Anil Shukla]

The 31 spinal cord segments correspond to each of these vertebrae: 8 cervical segments (the first cervical spinal cord segment is above the first cervical vertebra), 12 thoracic, 5 lumbar, 5 sacral, and 1 coccygeal. Each spinal cord segment has a pair of spinal nerves, one exiting on the right and another on the left side of the spinal cord between vertebrae to send and receive impulses to and from nerves in the rest of the body (such as skin, muscles, and various organs). Each spinal nerve (on the right and the left) divides into two major bundles of fibers (called a ramus), one toward the back (the dorsal primary ramus) and one toward the front (the ventral primary ramus).

During the first three months of development in the womb, the spinal cord of the human fetus extends the entire length of the vertebral canal. But by birth the spinal cord's conical end (the conus medullaris) usually occurs around the third lumbar vertebra. In adults the spinal cord occupies only the upper two-thirds of the vertebral canal, ending around the second lumbar vertebra. By adulthood, the paired spinal nerve roots exiting the lower spinal cord have grown long enough below the conus medullaris to exit well below the lower lumbar region to serve the legs and feet.

Although the 31 pairs of spinal nerves delineate different spinal cord segments, the spinal cord itself is one long, continuous, unitary structure, each segment merging into the next with little alteration of its internal structure. Nerve impulses pass up and down the length of the spinal cord seamlessly, along long tracts made up of numerous nerve fibers. The spinal cord's most critical smooth and unbroken connection is, of course, with the brain.

Finally, the entire central nervous system—the brain and the spinal cord—is protected by a cushion of fluid, the cerebrospinal fluid (CSF). While the skull and vertebral column provide the first line of defense against external injury, the CSF pillows these soft organs within their bony armor. The dura mater, a thick firm layer of dense connective tissue, lines the inner surface of the skull and vertebral canal. The spinal dura mater is shaped like a tube with periodic openings for the spinal nerves to emerge. Underneath the dura mater is the subarachnoid space within which the CSF circulates, providing the fluid cushion. The brain and spinal cord themselves are covered by a thin filmy layer called the pia mater, which is barely visible to the human eye but gives the brain, when exposed, its shiny appearance.

CSF is produced by the choroid plexus (thin, highly vascular tissue, repeatedly folded into tiny finger-like projections) of the lateral, third, and fourth ventricles of the brain. CSF is clear and colorless. Its glucose level is half that found in blood, and its protein level is normally extremely low. The volume of CSF ranges from 80 to 150 milliliters, and the choroid plexus produces enough to replace the full volume of CSF several times daily. The venous bloodstream absorbs old CSF to maintain a constant volume of fluid in the subarachnoid space during normal circumstances. As described in Chapter 2, laboratory and microscopic examination of CSF has been central to diagnostic evaluation of MS since the early 1900s.

CENTRAL NERVOUS SYSTEM CELLS

Each organ system in the human body has its own distinctive types of cells specialized to perform the specific functions of that particular organ. For example, the glomerular cells that conduct the filtration and cleansing work of kidneys differ significantly from the striated muscle cells that produce movement in arms and legs. The central nervous system does contain cell types present in other parts of the body. Examples include the cells that make up blood vessels (arteries, veins, and capillaries) and the cells circulating in blood, such as red blood cells (erythrocytes, which transport essential oxygen to tissues, including the brain and spinal cord) and white blood cells of various types (including granulocytes and lymphocytes, which attack infections and direct the immune response; see Chapter 4). But the cells that perform the complex functions of the central nervous system are unique and highly specialized. Different categories of cells have very specific roles.

The central nervous system has two primary categories of specialized cells: nerve cells, also known as neurons; and neuroglial cells, sometimes called simply glia or neuroglia, which come in a variety of types (Kiernan, 2009). Neurons perform the primary business of the central nervous system and are specialized to conduct and receive impulses and exchange signals with other neurons. Neuroglia, depending on their type (astrocytes, ependymal cells, microglia, and oligodendrocytes), perform various supportive functions to assist the neurons and police and repair central nervous system tissues.

The job of the neuron is rapid communication. Neurons specialize in sending and receiving electrical or chemical signals from other neurons. Neurons have a cell body, which contains its nucleus (see Figure 1.2). Most of the cytoplasm (substance of the cell outside of the nucleus but within the cell wall) of neurons is in extensions or processes of two types, dendrites and axons. Dendrites, which are typically short and branching, generally receive signals from other neurons. Most central nervous system neurons have several dendrites fanning out from the cell body. Some neurons have no axons but instead have multiple dendrites that both send and receive messages from other neurons (signals move in both directions).

In contrast, those neurons with axons have only one axon. Axons vary substantially in length depending on their location and role. Typically, signals

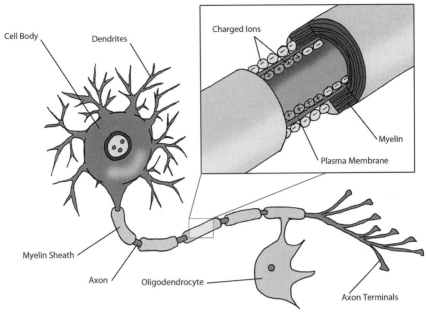

Figure 1.2. Neuron with Its Myelin Sheath. Neurons, or nerve cells, send and receive electrical or chemical signals to and from other neurons through their extensions: short branching dendrites; and long axons surrounded by myelin sheaths produced by oligodendrocytes. Gaps in the myelin sheath (nodes of Ranvier) and electrical gradients across the plasma membranes of axons facilitate rapid transmission of electrical impulses. [Anil Shukla]

transmitted along axons move away from the cell body, traveling in one direction. Axons vary in length. The axon of a motor neuron in the spinal cord serving a foot muscle can be nearly one meter long, while axons of other neurons are only 100 microns (one micron = one-millionth of a meter) in length.

Signals sent down axons terminate at a synapse, which is where nervous impulses pass to the target neuron or other cell, indicating what that cell should do. Specifically, at the synapse, the axon releases an electrical or chemical transmitter that is recognized by the receiving cell, which is either stimulated to or inhibited from performing a particular function. Persons move their legs, for instance, because signals speedily pass down the axons of multiple motor neurons and are received through synapses of their targeted striated muscle cells in the leg. All this happens so rapidly that the signals and muscle responses are virtually simultaneous.

Speed is essential. An electrical gradient between the inside and the outside of the axon facilitates this almost instantaneous passage of signals. Neuronal impulses are propagated or conducted along the surface of the axon's outer membrane, specifically on the plasma membrane (a double layer of phospholipid molecules, which has different types of protein molecules embedded within it). Some of the protein molecules create channels allowing inorganic chemical ions to pass in and out of the cell, including sodium (Na^+), potassium (K^+), and chloride (Cl^-). Each ion has either a positive or negative charge. In the fluid outside the cell, Na^+ and Cl^- are the most common ions; their charges balance out, to make this fluid neutral. Inside the cell, K^+ is most common, although organic anions (negative ions) of amino acids and proteins counterbalance the positive charge of the potassium ions. The plasma membrane's mesh is too fine to allow relatively large organic anions to pass through and exit the cell, and the protein molecule channels typically prevent movement of Na^+ into the cell.

As shown in the inset of Figure 1.2, this situation sets up an electrical gradient between the inside and the outside of the cell when the axon is at rest. The inside is slightly negatively charged (approximately −70 millivolt, mV) compared with the fluid outside the cell. However, when a nerve cell is stimulated, some of the protein molecules protecting the plasma membrane respond, allowing inorganic ions to flow across the membrane. The electrical gradient in a stimulated cell reverses to become slightly positive inside the cell (+40 mV) compared with the outside. This reversal of the electrical gradient is called the action potential or impulse, and it moves instantly down the axon carrying the signal to its ultimate target—a synapse with a muscle or some other type of cell. When the action potential reaches the synapse, the neuron releases its electrical or chemical transmitter that tells the receiving cell what to do.

GREY AND WHITE MATTER

Although the electrical action potential moves speedily down an axon, signaling needs to be virtually instantaneous. This is where the support cells, the neuroglia, come in: specifically a type of neuroglia called the oligodendrocyte. Among other activities, oligodendrocytes produce a protein sheath that surrounds the axon from near where it travels out from the cell body to just short of its terminal branching at the synapse (see Figure 1.2). This sheath is made of myelin protein. Oligodendrocytes produce the myelin sheath by winding thin layers of their plasma membrane around and around the axon, until the encased structure is many times the diameter of the axon alone. A single oligodendrocyte can wrap a myelin sheath around as many as 40 axons, and multiple adjacent oligodendrocytes contribute short sections to the sheath encasing a single axon.

The myelin sheath has a special feature that bolsters speedy conduction of the action potential. As shown in Figure 1.2, the sheath is not smooth and continuous along the full length of the axon. Instead, periodically tiny interruptions occur, at the places where the myelin sheath laid down by one oligodendrocyte abuts the segment supplied by its neighboring oligodendrocyte. These infinitesimal gaps are called nodes of Ranvier, and they are responsible for the rapidity of signal transmission down myelinated axons.

In myelinated axons, the ion movements described above that cause impulse conduction occur only at nodes of Ranvier. This means that the action potential jumps from node to node rather than having to travel the entire length of the axon. This jumping movement is called saltatory conduction, and it increases the speed of signaling significantly. Motor neuron axons, which are all myelinated, conduct impulses to skeletal muscle cells at 70–120 meters/second (Kiernan, 2009, 23). In contrast, nerve fibers relating to pain and temperature sensation and the sense of smell are unmyelinated, and their conduction velocities are only 0.5–2.5 meters/second.

Thus, the myelin protein sheaths produced by oligodendrocytes, which encase the axons of neurons, are essential to normal functioning of the central nervous system. A single axon and its myelin sheath are invisible to the human eye. However, in the central nervous system, many thousands of these nerve fibers travel together, each heading toward neighboring, interrelated destinations: for example, numerous motor neuron axons extend down the spinal cord to stimulate muscle cells that move the legs, feet, and toes. The myelin sheaths surrounding these thousands of neural axons appear whitish to the naked eye. Myelin accounts for about 70 percent of the dry weight of the central nervous system in mammals (Compston, Lassmann, and Smith, 2005, 466).

If one cuts open a cross-section of the human brain—or slices across a segment of the spinal cord—the tissues will have a consistent pattern, some parts appearing grayish and other parts whitish. The gray matter consists of neuron cell bodies, each with its nucleus, embedded within a microscopic meshwork of supporting neuroglia and the filamentous processes of neighboring neurons. The white matter consists of the axons of many thousands of neurons, encased in their myelin sheaths along with their supportive oligodendrocytes and other neuroglia. On an imaging study, such as a CT or MRI scan, these patterns of gray and white tissues appear prominently, delineating the anatomy of different sections of the central nervous system.

MS: A WHITE MATTER DISEASE

As shown in Figure 1.3, the primary lesions of MS are destruction of the myelin sheaths surrounding the axons of neurons with some injury to the axons themselves (Morales, Parisi, and Lucchinetti, 2006). Because of this myelin loss, MS is often called a white matter disease. Myelin destruction is most common in certain

Normal   ## MS

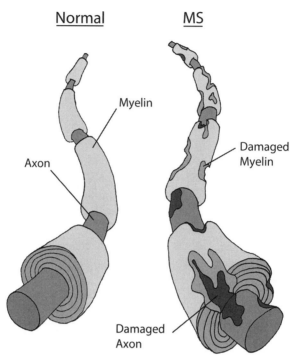

Myelin

Axon

Damaged
Myelin

Damaged
Axon

Figure 1.3. Damage to Myelin Sheaths and Axons in MS. The primary lesions of MS are destruction of myelin sheaths surrounding axons of neurons and damage or degeneration of the axons themselves. [Anil Shukla]

sections of the central nervous system, most notably the periventricular white matter deep within the brain, two critical regions of the brain (the cerebellum and the brain stem), the spinal cord, and the optic nerves. These locations, in turn, dictate the exact locations and nature of symptoms experienced by persons with MS.

Areas where the myelin is destroyed are known as plaques, and to the human eye they appear gray and translucent. The word sclerotic, which means hardened, was used to describe this appearance in the mid-1800s, when scientists, such as Robert Carswell and Edmé Vulpian, began noting specific lesions associated with a mysterious neurological disease (see Chapter 2, which recounts this history). The Parisian neurologist Jean-Martin Charcot first described MS systematically in 1868, and the name multiple sclerosis reflected the multiple sclerotic plaques found throughout the central nervous systems of deceased patients who had had the disease and underwent autopsy.

Under the microscope, the plaque has a very specific appearance. Most obvious is the myelin loss and damage to the underlying axon. In addition, areas surrounding the blood vessels that supply oxygen to the tissues show signs of inflammation, and astrocytes (a type of neuroglia cell that performs multiple different functions) form scars. Plaques undergo distinct stages, evolving from an early stage when the myelin is being actively destroyed to an inactive stage. Sometimes oligodendrocytes remyelinate denuded axons; in other instances, the plaque remains unmyelinated, and no oligodendrocytes populate the area. Immune system cells called macrophages consume and slowly digest the myelin basic protein released as myelin sheaths are destroyed. By the time a plaque becomes inactive, all the macrophages have disappeared, and primarily astrocytes remain. About 70 percent of persons with MS have plaques still populated by oligodendrocytes and extensive remyelination (Morales, Parisi, and Lucchinetti, 2006, 31). The other 30 percent have plaques with few oligodendrocytes and little remyelination. Remyelination restores the essential functional abilities of the axons.

What causes the damage to myelin sheaths remains under active investigation. As discussed in Chapter 4, many leading scientists believe that an autoimmune process occurs where the body's own immune cells attack myelin sheaths, but other scientists dispute this scenario. In any case, degeneration of myelin sheaths, along with associated axonal damage, impedes and slows the saltatory conduction of action potentials down the axons. Thus, nerves are unable to tell their target tissues what to do—and are unable to receive messages back—as quickly as before demyelination. This has serious consequences for communication back and forth among various nerves, up, down, and throughout the central nervous system. Damage that occurs at this microscopic level translates directly into the myriad symptoms experienced by persons with MS.

2

History of MS

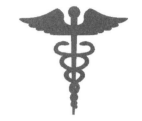

Sally Ann Jones, who is now in her mid-fifties, thinks her MS symptoms started when she was 19 years old. But she was not diagnosed with MS until her early thirties. "Starting long ago, I had weakness and numbness in my legs that would come and go," Mrs. Jones recalled. "Right after my son was born, the left side of my face went numb." The numbness disappeared after several months. Then one summer day, her small son started crying while playing across the street. When Mrs. Jones tried to run to reach his side, she could not move her legs. "My legs wouldn't run. All I could do was lope along." That problem eventually got better, too.

Over the years, Mrs. Jones periodically visited her primary care doctor to try to diagnose what was causing her many strange and ephemeral symptoms. Her doctor had few answers. At one appointment, "the doctor said I was exhausting myself by having two small children at home and going to my job. If I would just change my life style a bit, he said, I would get better." Finally, the primary care doctor "threw up his hands" and sent Mrs. Jones to a neurologist.

This happened in the 1960s, two decades before major advances in diagnosing MS. At that time, diagnoses were made primarily by taking careful clinical histories from patients, doing thorough physical examinations, and eliminating other possible diagnoses. The neurologist suggested that Mrs. Jones might have a pinched nerve and then said offhandedly, without further elaboration, "I don't think you have MS." This comment caught Mrs. Jones off guard. "I hardly knew what MS was. It was one of those poster diseases. I could picture somebody sitting in a wheelchair. I was elated not to have MS."

But four months later, Mrs. Jones returned to the neurologist. Her strange symptoms had persisted without relief. This time, the neurologist diagnosed MS. Mrs. Jones remembers him describing how he reached that conclusion. Because she had not yet died of a brain tumor—another possible diagnosis he had considered but not mentioned during her earlier visit—the neurologist reasoned that Mrs. Jones must have MS.

* * * * *

The story of how Mrs. Jones was diagnosed with MS parallels the history of how doctors finally recognized this complicated and perplexing disease. It took many years for scientists to link together the widely differing patterns of symptoms— the great variety of problems reported by patients and the lengthy, meandering time course—as representing a specific disease. In fact, some still question whether MS is a single disease rather than several closely related but distinct diseases. Broadly speaking, MS comes in differing patterns (types or variants), defined by the timing, pace, and extent of symptoms and disability (see Table 2.1). In the years before her diagnosis, Sally Ann Jones had relapsing-remitting MS: episodic

Table 2.1
Patterns of Multiple Sclerosis

Pattern	Description
Relapsing-remitting	Clear relapses (flares), followed by complete or partial recovery. Approximately 85 percent of MS cases at onset of disease symptoms.
Secondary progressive	Gradual worsening of MS symptoms without discrete flares or recovery. Follows initial relapsing-remitting disease pattern for most patients with that initial MS type.
Primary progressive	Continual worsening from time of MS onset, perhaps with occasional plateau or minor improvement of symptoms. Approximately 10 percent of MS cases.
Progressive relapsing	Continual worsening from time of MS onset, with clear relapses (flares) with marked worsening followed sometimes by partial resolution of relapse symptoms. Approximately 5 percent of MS cases.

flares of symptoms or problems followed by periods of remission (disappearance and absence of symptoms). After her diagnosis, her MS shifted gradually to the secondary progressive type, as her disability slowly worsened or progressed without periods of recovery.

This chapter examines three topics. First, it explores the history of how MS was finally recognized as a disease about 150 years ago. Second, it considers how ideas about what causes MS have evolved over time. Finally, this chapter reviews the history of approaches and technologies used to diagnose MS. If a 30-year-old Sally Ann Jones went to a neurologist today with the same set of symptoms and clinical history, she would have a very different diagnostic evaluation.

RECOGNIZING MS AS A DISEASE

In his comprehensive book *Multiple Sclerosis: The History of a Disease* (2005), the renowned Canadian neurologist and medical historian T. Jock Murray starts with a conundrum: many different conditions can cause weakness and its more extreme form, paralysis. Furthermore, sometimes this growing weakness progresses to paralysis slowly, over years or even decades. Doctors would need to observe patients for very long periods to track this progression. Beyond paralysis, many conditions might produce other key features of MS, such as vision problems, generalized fatigue, urinary incontinence, and cognitive difficulties (see Chapter 5). With the medical tools available in earlier centuries, how could doctors sort through these numerous different symptom patterns and varying courses of illness to describe a distinct and specific disease? Or, as Murray (2005, 19) asked, "What is a disease before it gets a name?"

While the biological factors that produce MS have likely existed for centuries, it is difficult to identify early cases of the disease. Disease and disability were viewed very differently hundreds of years ago than they are today. In sixteenth-century England, for example, the Elizabethan Prayer Book couched illness and infirmity in religious or theological terms as God's visitations (Starr, 1982, 35–36). Treatments or interventions by human healers, while worth trying, could work only with God's permission. In sixteenth- and seventeenth-century England, proper responses to accidents or disease involved searching the person's soul for moral culpability or fault.

The Virgin Lidwina, who was born in 1380 in Schiedam, Holland, and died in 1433, may represent the first documented case of MS, although religious fervor and mysticism shroud her story (Compston, Lassmann, and McDonald, 2005, 7; Murray, 2005, 21–26). One of nine children of a laborer father, she had been a healthy teenager. But Lidwina developed a series of physical ailments, some transitory, following a fall while skating on a frozen canal in 1396. She had difficulty walking without holding onto furniture and, at times, spent much of her days in bed. She became blind in one eye, experienced severe pains in her face and other parts of her body, developed weakness in one arm and one side of her face, and had some loss of sensation.

With frequent visits from her parish priest, Lidwina grew to believe she had been called to suffer for the sins of others. Starting in 1407, Lidwina began reporting supernatural visitations or ecstasies, visions involving participation in the Passion of Christ and encounters with saints. During these periods, her mobility and vision improved. Her piety and suffering attracted public notice, and many doctors came to consult on her case, although one prominent physician pronounced her incurable since her condition came directly from God. A cult coalesced around Lidwina, extolling her saintly virtues. In 1890, Pope Leo XIII canonized her as Saint Lidwina (her name is spelled various ways, including Lydwyna and Ludwine). She is the patron saint of sickness and of figure skating because of her teenage fall while skating on the frozen canal.

Whether the Virgin Lidwina truly is the first known case of MS remains controversial. Neurologists have debated reports of her various health problems and found aspects that are consistent with MS but also possibly with other medical conditions. Complicating this assessment is the mysticism pervading her story, the fervent religiosity of her behaviors, and the biological implausibility of some claims (an official testimonial produced by the municipality of Schiedam asserted she drank no fluids for seven years). Lidwina's bones were identified in 1947, and an analysis at a Dutch laboratory in 1957 found changes in the right arm and leg bones consistent with paralysis. Nonetheless, controversy remains about Lidwina's MS diagnosis.

In combing records from the next three centuries, cases occasionally arose that suggested MS, but most descriptions leave room for debate. One virtually certain case of relapsing-remitting MS (the patterns where disease symptoms come and go; see Table 2.1), which later evolved into secondary progressive disease, was Augustus d'Esté (1794–1848), grandson of King George III of England and cousin of Queen Victoria (Compston, Lassmann, and McDonald, 2005, 13–15; Murray, 2005, 32–41). Prince Augustus Frederick, Duke of Sussex, upset his father, George III, by secretly marrying Lady Augusta Murray in Rome. Because marriages of heirs to the British throne required the king's consent, which the prince had not received, George III annulled the marriage. The annulment made the couple's child, Augustus, illegitimate. Abandoned by the prince, his mother raised Augustus in England. Attempting to establish his formal ties to the monarchy, Augustus d'Esté later appealed to four kings, a prime minister, and the House of Lords, but he failed to win his case.

Starting in 1822 and for the rest of his life, d'Esté kept a diary where he documented a wide variety of symptoms that would come and go. On the first page of the diary he wrote about his vision blurring, worsening to the point where he could no longer read. Later his eyesight improved. This cycle, sometimes complicated by double vision, recurred several times. D'Esté also described episodes of leg numbness, walking difficulties, weakness, vertigo, bladder difficulties, impotence, and extreme heat sensitivity—all common problems of MS (see Chapter 5). The diaries documented various treatments prescribed by numerous medical attendants, including bleeding by leeches, rubbing of his legs with brushes, flannel bandages, courses of electricity, various herbs, strychnine, quinine, mercury, iron, cold water baths, horseback riding, walking in the Scottish highlands, sea bathing, a diet rich in beef steak and Madeira wines, and brandy and water. Treatments either failed or recoveries were brief, and d'Esté moved on to new rounds of symptoms, another medical consultant, and different attempts at cures.

In his diary, d'Esté wrote of his emotional ups and downs, his handwriting sometimes shaky and hard to read. In early adulthood, d'Esté had come across as arrogant, selfish, and argumentative. By the time of his death in 1848, his diary told a different story. When he sold his carriage, for example, he sent the money to relieve persons suffering from the Irish famine. D'Esté had grown deeply appreciative of his friends who would visit since he could no longer easily leave his rooms. He became sensitive to the health concerns of others as he persisted in doggedly confronting his recurrent medical problems.

While the Virgin Lidwina's condition was seen as an act of God in the 1400s, by the time of Augustus d'Esté in the 1800s, perceptions of physical ailments and their root causes had changed dramatically. Dawning understanding of human anatomy and how various organs worked in the body—as well as what might go awry with organ system functioning—had deepened by the early nineteenth century. Some physicians consulted by d'Esté believed his malady originated in his nerves, although his doctors had little appreciation of what caused his damaged nerve functioning.

The first description by a physician of a likely MS case occurred in Paris in 1824, with publication of *Maladies de la moelle épinière* (*Disorders of the Spinal Cord*) by the 28-year-old Charles Prosper Ollivier d'Angers (1796–1845) (Murray, 2005, 62–64). Ollivier described the anatomy and functioning of the spinal cord and various disorders relating to spinal cord pathology, such as cysts and spina bifida (a congenital defect in which the bony encasement of the spinal cord does not close properly, producing paralysis). Ollivier's treatise described a probable case of relapsing-remitting MS—a man whose symptoms likely started at age 17 and included periodic bouts of leg weakness, fatigue, distorted sensations, bladder difficulties, hand clumsiness, and other problems. Ollivier suggested that infection caused the spinal cord damage, leading him to recommend bleeding and placement of leeches across the man's upper chest and back. The man lived with his disease for 29 years.

Scottish physician Robert Carswell (1793–1857), who had a remarkable talent for drawing, produced the first illustrations of how MS damages nerves (Murray, 2005, 66–71). Carswell spent 1822 and 1823 in Paris and Lyons, France, drawing specimens from autopsies. He gathered these illustrations, along with sketches from Scotland and elsewhere, into an atlas or collection of drawings published in 1838, *Pathological Anatomy: Illustrations of the Elementary Forms of Disease.* The finely detailed illustrations, some etched directly onto lithographic stones for printing, showed the spinal cord of a paralyzed patient who had died and undergone autopsy. Describing the condition as a "peculiar diseased state," Carswell illustrated discoloration and hardening of the white matter, fresh lesions (abnormal areas) and old scars, and atrophy (or thinning) of the spinal cord.

Thus, starting with Ollivier and Carswell, the first half of the nineteenth century in Europe was a fertile time and place as physicians and scientists, primarily in France, Germany, and Great Britain, drew closer to recognizing and describing the disease MS. Physicians became increasingly aware that a progressive condition existed that affected young adults, involved the spinal cord, and caused softening of tissues and multiple harder grey patches in the central nervous system. The microscope opened new understanding as scientists using this tool identified different types of cells and structures in the nervous system. In 1866, Edmé Vulpian (1826–1887), the eminent French physician-scientist and expert in microscopy, first employed the phrase "sclérose en plaque disséminée" (hardening in multiple plaques).

In 1868, the Parisian neurologist Jean-Martin Charcot (1825–1893; see Figure 2.1) gave three lectures that presented, for the first time, a comprehensive clinical description, along with evidence about central nervous system damage, that identified MS as a disease (Compston, Lassmann, and McDonald, 2005, 26–29; Murray, 2005, 103–130). Paris at that time was a hub of medical discovery, and Charcot's observations were aided by his research at the massive Salpêtrière institution. That huge building—originally a munitions factory and arsenal (its name comes from saltpeter, an ingredient of gunpowder) before neighbors complained about repeated explosions—had become home to 5,000 poor women who were elderly, sick, mentally incompetent, or disabled, without families to care for them at home.

Along with his colleague Vulpian, also assigned to Salpêtrière duty, Charcot methodically assessed these women, classifying each by her condition and sorting them into logical categories. Assisted by various students and collaborators, they

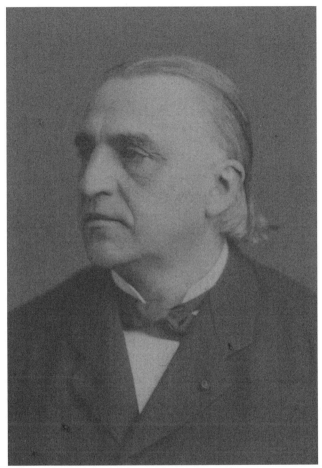

Figure 2.1. Jean-Martin Charcot. Parisian neurologist Jean-Martin Charcot (1825–1893) provided the first clinical description of MS as a specific disease. [The Boston Medical Library in the Francis A. Countway Library of Medicine]

methodically built extensive case files on each woman and, after the woman's death, linked autopsy information and studies of the diseased tissues under the microscope with descriptions of their clinical symptoms, behaviors, and histories. Thus, Salpêtrière offered a ripe environment for the first systematic description of MS: many patients, long-term observations, the ability to examine living patients clinically and their tissues after death, and careful scientists who employed logical organizational methods to compare, group, and describe cases.

In his three lectures in 1868 on "la sclérose en plaque disséminée," Charcot laid essential groundwork for defining a disease. Foremost, he described the disorder, identifying features that distinguished it from other conditions. These detailed descriptions would allow other physicians to recognize and diagnose MS in their own patients. Furthermore, based on his own microscopic examinations and those of his colleague Vulpian, Charcot described the pathology of the disease: the destruction of myelin and preservation of axons (see Chapters 1 and 4). He related this pathology seen under the microscope to the symptoms that patients experience. Finally, Charcot outlined how the disease progresses, sketching what would be later recognized as relapsing-remitting and secondary progressive MS patterns (see Table 2.1).

Charcot admitted that he did not know what causes MS. In later years, he recognized that the disease occurs primarily among women, often starting in early adulthood. He had few suggestions about treatment, appropriately dismissing common therapies of the day—such as arsenic, strychnine, belladonna, and potassium bromide—as of little use. Despite this, Charcot's lectures, translated and disseminated across Europe, North America, and Australia, led to recognition of MS as a disease and sparked considerable interest in finding ways to diagnose, understand, and treat the condition. Starting in the 1870s, MS was increasingly diagnosed in patients around the world. This previously unrecognized disease grew to be acknowledged as the most common neurological condition affecting young adults.

EVOLVING IDEAS ABOUT WHAT CAUSES MS

The next two chapters discuss current thinking about what causes MS. Considerable strides in understanding these causes have occurred over the last 150 years—and have advanced leagues beyond the act of God views of illness in general that dominated the time of the Virgin Lidwina. D'Esté attributed his vision loss to stress on his eyesight caused by holding back tears at the funeral of a dear friend. Despite recent scientific discoveries, however, ideas about causes of MS are still evolving. The exact cause of MS remains unknown today.

When Jean-Martin Charcot described MS as a disease, he acknowledged not knowing the cause. Other physicians at the time suggested that blood vessel problems cause MS, but Charcot disagreed. Although he noted that MS sometimes started after persons had an infection, Charcot also dismissed infection as a possible cause. Over ensuing years, numerous theories about what causes MS have held sway. In his 1882 textbook on spinal diseases, British physician Sir Byrom Bramwell (1847–1931) conjectured that many cases of MS occurred after some injury, such as trauma to the head or spine, or after persons were exposed to wet or cold conditions. In 1903, Bramwell delineated varying geographical patterns of disease occurrence, noting higher MS rates in northern Scotland compared with New York. However, Bramwell did not link these geographic differences to specific causes (see Chapter 3).

In 1884, Pierre Marie (1853–1940), a French physician and student of Charcot, published an article linking MS with infectious diseases (Murray, 2005, 176–180). After enumerating other causes he viewed as well accepted, including cold exposure, trauma, overwork, and every manner of excessive behavior, Marie asserted that infectious causes were by far more common. As noted in Chapters 3 and 4, some possible role for infectious agents remains on today's lists of contributing causes to MS. Although Marie steadfastly endorsed an infectious cause, he did not target specific microbes. Living during a period of exciting discoveries about bacteria and infectious agents—the same era as French bacteriologist and chemist Louis Pasteur (1822–1895), British surgeon Joseph Lister (1827–1912, who introduced antiseptic techniques), and German bacteriologist Robert Koch (1843–1910)—Marie suggested treating MS using therapies that targeted infections, such as iodide of potassium or sodium and mercury.

In the late nineteenth and early twentieth centuries, different experts held varying opinions about the cause of MS. In addition to trauma and infectious causes, other possibilities—now discredited—included vascular disorders, metabolic problems, constipation, physical and mental stress, excessive sexual activity, heavy alcohol consumption, exposures to toxins (such as copper, lead, or zinc), heat or cold exposures, seizures during childhood, and selected occupations (such as woodworking, farming, working with aniline dyes or phosphorus, and jobs involving certain animals). In the early decades of the twentieth century, when the psychoanalytic theories of Sigmund Freud (1856–1939) dominated psychiatric discourse, American psychoanalyst Smith Ely Jelliffe (1866–1945) suggested that MS plaques formed in the brain because of repressed emotions, with plaques targeting sites of the brain affected by emotional repression. He advocated treating MS with psychoanalysis. MS experts at a 1921 meeting rejected Jelliffe's theory.

By the 1950s, experts had eliminated most early theories about the causes of MS. Interest coalesced around contributions of some infectious agent, genetic linkages, and malfunctioning of the body's immune system. Chapters 3 and 4 describe these possibilities. Here suffice it to say that, despite dramatic growth in understanding within such fields as genetics and immunology, science in these areas is still evolving. For individual persons, multiple factors might conspire together, contributing to patients developing MS. In other words, no single cause may ever be found. This part of the MS story does not yet have a conclusive ending and awaits new discoveries.

EVOLVING APPROACH FOR DIAGNOSING MS

The factors that contributed to MS not being recognized for centuries as a distinct disease—highly variable symptoms, waxing and waning impairments, long time course, and features similar to other conditions—also affect the ability to diagnose MS, with certainty, in individual patients such as Sally Ann Jones. The neurologist who ultimately diagnosed Mrs. Jones relied exclusively on observing her: on her clinical history, which covered many years, and physical examination. In that way, the neurologist followed the teachings of Jean-Martin Charcot, the Parisian neurologist who first explicitly described MS, who noted, "Let someone say of a doctor that . . . he is an observer, a man who knows how to see, this is perhaps the greatest compliment one can make" (Murray, 2005, 135).

Even today with sophisticated imaging technologies and other diagnostic tools (see Chapter 5), the clinical history and physical examination remain the mainstay standard of MS diagnosis. Despite this, one significant disadvantage of the clinical diagnosis of MS is that it takes time: persons must wait to see how their symptoms evolve. Anxious to begin today's MS treatments (see Chapter 6), some persons with possible diagnoses of MS may not want to wait for this definitive diagnosis.

Neurologists starting with Charcot developed specific physical examination procedures for diagnosing MS, based on understanding the anatomy of the central nervous system and the way specific nerves function by making muscles and other bodily structures respond. These physical examination maneuvers involve testing patients' sensation, strength, reflexes, walking, vision, and various other aspects of neurological functioning. Sometimes, early neurologists used primitive means to assist diagnosis. The French physician d'Angers mentioned above, who explored spinal cord disorders, noted that some persons could not get out when placed into a hot tub of water—heat sapped all their strength (Murray, 2005, 64). Since some persons with MS are remarkably sensitive to heat, this hot bath test was later used to support the diagnosis of MS.

Joseph-François-Félix Babinski (1857–1932), a Parisian physician and student of Charcot, published a brief article in an 1896 medical journal describing a physical reflex suggesting central nervous system dysfunction: when the outer or lateral part of the sole of the foot is stimulated (such as by stroking or drawing a blunt, narrow instrument along its length), toes of normal individuals curl under, while the great toe of many persons with MS flexes upward and other toes fan outward. Testing for this so-called Babinski reflex remains part of neurological examinations today.

Even with extensive physical examinations, diagnosis of MS was far from perfect. Because other diseases can have similar physical findings, errors in diagnosis occurred fairly often and were detected only after time passed and patients developed signs or symptoms of other disorders. Through the mid-twentieth century, frustrated neurologists sought more specific tests to definitively diagnose MS. The first such test involved analysis of the cerebrospinal fluid (CSF), the colorless liquid that bathes and circulates throughout the sac protecting the brain and spinal cord. To obtain CSF for testing, physicians in the early 1900s devised a technique called the lumbar puncture. While patients lay on their sides, physicians inserted a long, hollow needle between the third and fourth vertebrae in the lumbar area of the spine, puncturing the sac protecting the spinal cord (which in adults ends well above the third lumbar vertebra so could not be damaged) and extracting a small amount of CSF for analysis. Lumbar punctures were originally used to test for syphilis in the CSF, but soon neurologists started applying the same approach to examine CSF for indicators of MS.

The CSF of persons with MS shows higher numbers of white blood cells (cells typically involved in immune responses; see Chapter 4) and higher-than-typical amounts of protein, especially myelin basic protein. In the 1940s, a new laboratory technique called electrophoresis offered opportunities to better understand other compounds floating in the CSF that could indicate specific types of diseases. Electrophoresis involves subjecting CSF (or other fluids or gels) to electrical currents and then watching how suspended particles move in response. Characteristic patterns of movement or migration identify specific types of compounds. In the case of the CSF of MS patients, researchers were especially interested in compounds called gamma globulins: antibodies produced by immune cells in the blood and other bodily fluids. With the dawning suspicion that an immune disorder might contribute to MS, researchers reasoned that gamma globulins might appear different in the CSF of MS patients than in other individuals.

During 20 years of research on CSF samples, scientists used electrophoresis to identify specific patterns of an antibody called immunoglobulin G suggestive of MS. They finally found a so-called oligoclonal pattern, in which specific immune globulins migrated together to produce several closely spaced bands on the electrophoresis filter paper (see Figure 5.4). (Olig means few, and clonal in this context means a group of replicas of some large molecule, such as an antibody.) Thus, one of the first scientific tests for MS—still used today—involves performing a lumbar puncture and subjecting the patient's CSF to microscopic study (looking for white blood cells), laboratory analysis (looking for myelin basic protein), and electrophoresis (looking for oligoclonal or several closely spaced bands of immune globulins).

Lumbar punctures, however, pose some hazards for patients, are uncomfortable, and can produce severe headaches that last several days. Therefore, despite this scientific advance, neurologists continued searching for less invasive tests to assist in diagnosing MS. X-rays, discovered in 1895 by German physicist Wilhelm Conrad Roentgen (1845–1923) while experimenting with cathode-ray tubes, were better at showing bones than soft structures, such as the brain and the spinal cord. Seventy years later, major advances in X-rays improved their sensitivity for this purpose. Computerized axial tomography (CAT), developed in the 1970s, involves rotating repeated X-ray beams around an object, such as the head, to determine the density of the tissues. Now called simply CT (computerized tomography) scanning, this technique produces clear pictures of soft tissues, including the brain.

Although neurologists were initially excited by thinking that CT scanning could assist MS diagnoses, their enthusiasm waned as they experimented with this new technology. The remarkable images produced by CT could not reliably identify MS plaques in the brain or spinal cord. Most individuals with definite MS according to their clinical diagnoses nonetheless had normal CT scans. CT was helpful for eliminating certain other potential causes of neurological symptoms, such as brain tumors, but it was not perfect in finding the brain lesions of MS.

The major advance for MS diagnosis came with development of magnetic resonance imaging (MRI) in the early 1980s: the first brain MRI occurred in 1981. MRI does not involve X-rays (thus sparing patients from the dangers of radiation exposure). Instead, while patients lie in the strong magnetic field of an MRI scanning machine, radio waves flip the spin of hydrogen nuclei in the water within their bodily tissues. When the nuclei relax back, they emit another radio wave, which the MRI machine detects and its computer uses to produce images of tissues in remarkable detail. Some have likened MRI images to crisp, precise black-and-white photographs of anatomy, all taken from outside the body. Brains and spinal cords of MS patients that appear completely normal in CT scans can demonstrate multiple MS lesions or plaques in MRI images (see Figure 5.3).

Despite its immense benefits, MRI does not render perfectly accurate diagnoses of MS. New MRI techniques, such as magnetization transfer imaging (MTI) and diffusion-tensor MRI (DT-MRI), might improve the ability of MRI to detect subtle lesions. Until then, as described in Chapter 5, neurologists sometimes use CSF analyses and other tests to provide more evidence to confirm MS diagnoses. As with virtually every aspect of this perplexing disease, only time will tell if an individual person with new symptoms and an MRI suggestive of MS really has the disease. Similarly to practices in Charcot's day 150 years ago, an absolutely definitive diagnosis of MS requires time and careful observation.

* * * * *

Sometimes people debate whether they would want to know if they have an incurable disease. Might they be happier not knowing since nothing can be done to cure them? How did Sally Ann Jones feel about this?

Mrs. Jones had had symptoms since age 19 that made her worried enough to go to the doctor over and over again and—even more importantly—were making it hard to care for her young family and do her job. She wanted to know what was happening to her, what was causing her odd sensations and troubling physical problems. She wanted to know if there was anything that could make her better. But when the neurologist told her she had MS, it came as a shock.

"I was afraid to go home," said Mrs. Jones, recalling that day.

I was afraid to tell my mother because I thought she would fall to pieces. I was afraid to tell anybody. I was afraid to tell myself. So I got in my car and drove around for a while. Thought about driving off the bridge. Thought about my children and husband and the only thing I knew about MS, which was to be in a wheelchair. How old was I? Thirty-three or so, and I had had MS for many many years but not known it.

Mrs. Jones went to the home of an older woman who had been her mentor in college and her friend for many years.

I stayed for about three hours and cried. I paced around. I tried to decide what to do. Then I knew I had to get on with things. I telephoned and told my mother, who didn't cry. Then I went home. Oh, I'll never forget this. The boys were playing basketball in the driveway when my husband came in and asked me what the doctor had said. I told him, and my husband sort of sighed. Then he said, "At least we know what it is. Now we can deal with it." So that was it.

For Mrs. Jones, knowing her diagnosis put to rest years of uncertainty and allowed her and her family to move on. They still had to deal with uncertainty. But at least what caused that uncertainty now had a name.

3

MS in Populations around the World

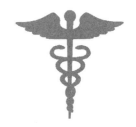

Lester Goodall was surprised when he learned he had MS. He does not fit the most common profile for the disease. Mr. Goodall is male and was in his early fifties when diagnosed. Like the late father of First Lady Michelle Obama, Fraser Robinson, who had MS, Mr. Goodall is African American. He has another major health condition, diabetes, which can cause neurological problems. But there were important clues. His older sister was diagnosed with MS many years earlier. In addition, Mr. Goodall was born and raised in Boston, Massachusetts, which is in New England, a northern region of the United States. Rates of MS typically rise with increasing distance from the equator, as regions get progressively cooler and receive lower intensity sunlight year-round.

The MS diagnosis did explain some things that had troubled Mr. Goodall for several years. One of his greatest pleasures had been throwing darts competitively in the Patriot Dart League on Wednesday evenings in Boston pubs. "I'd pick up my darts, trying to get the right position with my figures, but I couldn't," Mr. Goodall recalled.

> I'd stand on the white line, preparing to throw my dart and lose my balance
> with my next step. I thought maybe my diabetes was acting up. Or maybe
> I'd had too much to drink. When you throw a good shot with your dart,

you always take a little sip of your drink. If it's a bad shot, you take a little sip of your drink, too! I thought maybe the alcohol was making my diabetes and blood sugar go way out of control.

This is certainly a possible explanation for his physical unsteadiness.

Then another strange thing happened. "My vision went haywire," Mr. Goodall recounted. "It was like someone had taken the contrast on a TV and turned it down as dull as they could. I couldn't see the contrasts. So I went to my doctor.

"They put me through all of these tests. I found out that MS is diagnosed through a process of elimination. Finally the doctor told me I had MS." From that point on, "I changed some things. I got control of my diabetes, and I stopped drinking all alcohol. I couldn't throw darts any more. But I stayed with the Patriot League and became manager of the dart team."

Mr. Goodall is still trying to understand why he got MS. "My sister is older than me. She'd had MS for a long time and didn't know it. I think about the two of us, what we share that could relate to MS. Of course, there's genetics, and we both had chickenpox. Maybe it's the herpesvirus, which causes chickenpox and incubates over years within you afterward." Admitting that he's not a scientist—"a little knowledge makes me dangerous!"—Mr. Goodall favors his virus hypothesis.

* * * * *

Epidemiology is the study of patterns of diseases across different populations and groups of people. It builds upon the assumption that diseases do not occur randomly. Instead, diseases occur at higher rates among persons with some underlying trait or factor that makes them more likely to get the disease. The converse is also true: persons without those risk factors are less likely to develop the disease. Thus, by understanding the epidemiology of a disease, scientists can begin to hone in on the underlying risk factors or patient attributes and possibly identify potential causes of the illness.

Starting with Jean-Martin Charcot, who first described MS systematically (see Chapter 2), scientists began trying to identify personal and environmental factors associated with higher or lower rates of MS in various populations or groups of people. Failures to recognize and diagnose MS complicated epidemiology studies during the late nineteenth and early twentieth centuries. Much of this work relied on reports of causes of death by vital statistics registries, governmental agencies that record births and deaths.

By the mid-1900s, researchers had described the north-south gradient in MS deaths in North America and Europe: higher numbers of MS-related deaths occur as one moves farther away from the equator. The same pattern emerged among persons with European ancestry living in Australia, with MS rates increasing with growing distance from the equator. In addition, epidemiologists found that, while MS was recognized among Europeans, it was not found within indigenous populations in other parts of the world, such as Africa and Asia.

The distinctive geographic distribution of MS around the globe produced two lines of speculation. First, the concentration of MS among persons of northern European heritage raised conjectures about the role of genetics—inherited traits passed from parents to children—in the susceptibility for MS. Perhaps Europeans had genes that predisposed their offspring to developing MS, while persons from other racial groups did not. Second, the pattern of increasing MS rates with greater distance from the equator suggested that temperate climates or some systematic environmental exposure might contribute to the development of MS. Possibilities included a virus more common in cooler regions or even lower sunlight intensity. These intriguing observations have provided starting points for many epidemiological studies of MS, which like so much else about this disease, continue to uncover more mysteries than definitive solutions.

This chapter describes the patterns of MS in the United States and around the world. The chapter then looks at the several possible contributors to MS suggested by the epidemiologic studies: genetics or the inheritance of traits from one's parents; and environmental factors, including viruses and levels of sunlight exposure. Before starting, it is important to consider Mr. Goodall's hypothesis from his mini-epidemiological study within his own family where two siblings have MS. Mr. Goodall wondered about a role for the herpesvirus that causes chickenpox (specifically *Human herpesvirus 3*, also called *varicella*), which can reactivate years later to cause shingles. As described below, scientists have examined whether various different viruses could cause MS. So far, no definitive proof confirms that this happens, although several viruses have generated interest along these lines. Researchers have investigated Mr. Goodall's candidate—the chickenpox herpesvirus—without confirming a link to MS.

PATTERNS OF MS IN THE UNITED STATES

According to the National Institute of Neurological Disorders and Stroke (NINDS, 2009), no one knows precisely how many persons in the United States have MS. NINDS estimates the number at between 250,000 and 350,000, with approximately 200 new cases diagnosed weekly. Other estimates range as high as 400,000 Americans. Rates of MS in the population are five times higher in temperate northern states (such as Massachusetts, where Mr. Goodall was born) than in more tropical southern regions. Overall, the risk of developing MS among Americans is less than one-tenth of one percent (0.1 percent).

MS symptoms rarely begin before age 15 or after age 60, although new cases in young children and elderly individuals can occur. The age and sex distribution at first diagnosis varies by type of MS (Birnbaum, 2006, 111–112). As described in Chapter 5 (also see Table 2.1), relapsing-remitting MS is the most common form, present in about 85 percent of persons newly diagnosed with MS. Relapsing-remitting MS usually appears between 15 and 50 years of age, with two to three times more women than men. Despite this predominance among women, there is no evidence of a relationship between childbearing or the number of pregnancies and the development of relapsing-remitting MS. Primary progressive MS, which occurs in about 10 percent of newly diagnosed individuals, is typically identified between ages 30 and 60 years, with equal numbers of men and women. The rarest form of MS (progressive relapsing MS) has similar age and sex patterns as primary progressive MS.

MS occurs primarily among individuals of northern European ancestry. White persons are more than twice as likely to develop MS as are individuals of other races. MS is very uncommon among Native Americans, Asians, and African blacks. Many African Americans have white European ancestors, which may be the source of their genetic susceptibility to MS. This is likely the situation for Mr. Goodall, who correctly observed that white Americans far outnumber black Americans with MS.

In 1999, the National Multiple Sclerosis Society (NMSS) approved a study to survey persons with MS living throughout the United States to examine their demographic characteristics, treatment choices and outcomes, and other factors (Minden et al., 2006). Named after Sonya Slifka, who had immigrated to the United States from Latvia in the 1920s and was diagnosed with MS in 1948, the study showed that the majority of Americans with MS are women, white, and not Hispanic (see Table 3.1). (Mrs. Slifka's son Robert, who chaired the NMSS Board of Directors, contributed $1 million to this study in honor of his mother, who he said had an awe-inspiring stubbornness to continue being involved and active, despite her significant disability.)

MS AROUND THE WORLD

MS is very rare in many parts of the world. For instance, no Gypsies, Eskimos, or Bantus (persons living in Sub-Saharan Africa) are known to have MS; native Indians of North and South America, Japanese, and other Asian populations have extraordinarily low rates of MS (NINDS, 2009). While MS occurs among persons of European ancestry in Australia and New Zealand, with rising rates with increasing distance from the equator (see Figure 3.1), it is rare among

Table 3.1
Sex, Age, Race, and Ethnicity of Persons with MS Compared with the General Population in the United States

Characteristic	Persons with MS	General U.S. Population
Sex		
Female	77%	51%
Male	23	49
Age in years		
18–24	0.3	6
25–34	6	14
35–44	22	16
45–54	38	14
55–64	25	9
65–74	7	7
75+	2	6
Race		
White	88	79
African American	5	13
Other	8	11
Ethnicity		
Not Hispanic	96	87
Hispanic	4	13

Adapted from Minden et al. 2006. Comparisons with the general population come from the U.S. Census Bureau. Numbers within some characteristics may not add to 100% because of rounding error.

Aborigines of Australia and the Maoris of New Zealand. Efforts to count the numbers of persons living with MS worldwide are complicated by difficulties in identifying cases and ensuring accuracy of diagnoses. Epidemiologists have studied Europe most extensively, along with North America (Canada and the United States). This focus is justified by the relatively high frequency of MS among northern Europeans.

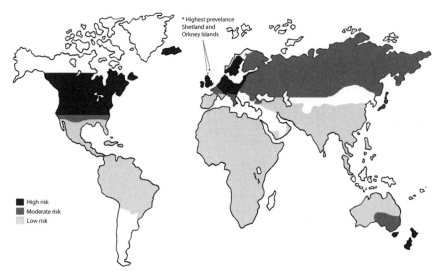

*Highest prevalence
Shetland and
Orkney Islands

High risk
Moderate risk
Low risk

Figure 3.1. Rates of MS by Geographic Region. This map shows the level of risk of developing MS in populations around the world. The risk of having MS increases in populations living farther from the equator, especially among those with northern European ancestry. [Anil Shukla]

The prevalence (percentage of population with a disease) of MS across Europe is estimated at 83 persons per 100,000 (0.083 percent), with a two-to-one ratio of women to men (Pugliatti et al., 2006). More than 200 epidemiological studies of MS have quantified prevalence rates in different European countries and regions. But differing methods and approaches for identifying cases of MS complicate comparisons of rates across studies and thus countries. Examples of the prevalence (per 100,000 persons) across European countries (and regions) include 187 in southeast Scotland; 168 in northern Ireland; 154 in Sweden; 127 in Germany; 122 in Denmark; 107 in Cambridgeshire, England; 58 in northern Spain; 53 in central Italy; 50 in France; and 39 in Greece. These numbers represent statistical estimates, and they are therefore not numerically precise. Nevertheless, a decreasing north-to-south gradient in the prevalence of MS is generally apparent, although there are some specific regions that present exceptions to these trends.

As shown in Figure 3.1, the Orkney and Shetland islands, off the northern coast of Scotland, have been thought to have one of the highest frequencies of MS within Europe (Compston and Confavreux, 2005, 82–83). Many of the Scottish epidemiologic studies, however, are now decades old. In 1974, an estimated 309 persons per 100,000 (approximately 0.31 percent) Orkney Island residents had MS, while in comparison, roughly 0.14 percent of the residents of

Aberdeen, a city on the eastern shore of Scotland south of the Orkney Islands, had MS. In recent years, the difference in MS rates between these northeastern Scottish islands and the rest of the United Kingdom has diminished somewhat, perhaps because of greater identification of MS cases in other parts of the country. Nonetheless, the striking findings of high prevalence of MS in the relatively small Orkney and Shetland Islands is viewed as supporting the role of heredity in the susceptibility for MS.

Few epidemiological studies have examined MS rates in the Middle East. Given the diverse geographic and ethnic origins of its population, MS studies in Israel have provided helpful insight into possible contributory factors, including genetics (Compston and Confavreux 2005, 93, 99). In one study, Jewish Israelis with European or American heritage had an MS prevalence of 0.064 percent (64 cases per 100,000 population). Arab Israelis had an MS prevalence of 0.019 percent (19 cases per 100,000 population). As described below, migration studies of various populations in Israel suggest that both genetics and environmental attributes might contribute to the development of MS.

GENETICS AND MS

When trying to identify causes of diseases, epidemiologic studies often run headlong into the long-standing nature-versus-nurture debate: are differences in the occurrence of diseases across populations caused by nature (biology, heredity, and genetic inheritance) or by nurture (physical and social environments)? Epidemiologic findings relating to race and MS within families, such as Mr. Goodall and his sister, strongly suggest that inherited genetic factors might contribute to an individual's likelihood of developing MS. In contrast, geographic patterns closely tracking cooler climates and lesser sunshine intensity raise speculation about potential environmental causes. It is also possible that both nature and nurture contribute to the likelihood of developing MS. The clinical heterogeneity of MS further complicates this debate.

Studies of MS patterns within families, where parents pass their genetic traits to their children and siblings share these genetic factors, provide good evidence that genes play some role—at least in increasing the risks of developing MS. In the U.S. population, the risk of developing MS is less than one-tenth of one percent (0.1 percent). However, the risk rises to 1–3 percent for persons with a first-degree relative (parent, sibling, or child) with MS (NINDS, 2009). Even more striking, if one identical twin has MS, the second identical twin has a 30-percent chance of developing MS (identical twins have identical genes, inherited from their parents). For fraternal twins (who do not have identical genes), the likelihood of MS is 4 percent (close to that of other siblings) when the other twin has the disease.

A major challenge confronting family studies is disentangling nature versus nurture effects. For instance, siblings who grew up in the same household share not only genes but also their social and physical environments: does biology or environment cause the higher risks of developing MS when a sibling gets the disease? To tease apart these issues, one strategy involves looking at family members who do not share their genetic inheritance. Examples include stepbrothers or stepsisters who grew up alongside their biologically unrelated sibling with MS or adopted children of parents with MS.

Epidemiologists have studied series of stepsiblings, half-siblings, and adopted children and demonstrated clearly that genetics—not the environment—determines the likelihood of developing MS when a biological relative has the disease. For instance, a study of 1,201 nonbiological relatives of persons with MS found only one case of MS. If results for first-degree, biological relatives had applied, 25 of these 1,201 individuals should have had MS (Sadovnick, 2006, 20). The finding of one case among the 1,201 (around 0.1 percent) represents roughly the rate of MS in the general population. Thus, although the environment likely plays some role in susceptibility to MS, environmental effects are probably not localized within the mini-environments of individual family households. Instead, environmental effects relate more broadly to populations and regions.

While family studies suggest an important role for genetic inheritance in susceptibility for MS, they also highlight the complexities of any potential relationship. If genes completely determine who will get MS, then both twins in pairs of identical twins should develop the disease. But this does not happen: only 30 percent of identical twins of persons with MS get symptoms of the disease.

Laboratory analyses of blood from persons with and without MS suggest that more than one gene is likely involved in determining the susceptibility of developing MS. In particular, researchers have examined genetic patterns of individuals with MS and found certain genetic markers are more frequent among those with MS than in persons without the disease. Researchers have focused particular attention on genetically determined proteins on blood cells that influence the immune system: human leukocyte antigen (HLA), encoded by the major histocompatibility complex region on chromosome 6. HLA patterns of persons with MS often differ from those of persons without MS, suggesting genetic differences between these two groups. Studies of Americans with MS have found three different HLAs, indicating three different genes on chromosome 6, that occur more frequently among persons with MS than in other individuals. However, not all persons with MS have these typical HLA patterns. Assessments of HLA patterns are therefore unhelpful in making a diagnosis of MS.

Other research has identified additional genes, involving chromosomes 2, 3, 7, 11, 17, and 19, as well as the X chromosome, that might contribute to developing MS (NINDS, 2009). However, no one has yet found strong and definitive relationships between individual genes and susceptibility of MS. Current thinking holds that multiple genes might affect a person's risk of MS, but each individual gene makes only a modest contribution. Different genes may also interact with other genes to heighten a person's risk. As with so much else about the disease, more research must explore the role of different genes in causing MS.

VIRUSES, ENVIRONMENTAL FACTORS, AND MS

As noted above (see Figure 3.1), rates of MS are five times higher in cooler climates, such as those of northern United States, Canada, and northern Europe, than in more tropical regions. One additional intriguing observation comes from migration studies—epidemiological studies of persons who move from one region to another. Migration studies support the possibility that environmental factors might contribute to development of MS and that persons have MS (or the predisposition to get the disease) for many years before symptoms appear.

Migration studies from different parts of the world have generally reached similar conclusions. If young people move from a high-MS region to a low-MS region before age 15, then their chances of acquiring MS become similar to those of persons in the low-MS region. The opposite also applies. When young people move from low-MS regions to high-MS regions before age 15, then their risk of developing the disease rises to that of the high-MS area. These findings suggest that something in the environment might either increase the likelihood of MS—or protect persons from getting MS—and that age 15 (around the time of puberty) is the critical moment for either raising or lowering the risk of MS. When individuals move after age 15, they keep the same risk of developing MS as in the area where they grew up (NINDS, 2009).

Migration studies from Israel have highlighted both potential genetic and environmental contributors to MS (Compston and Confavreux, 2005, 99). Israeli immigrants from northern Europe (Ashkenazi) have higher MS prevalence rates than do those from Asia and Africa (Shepardis). The age at immigration, however, has strong effects on MS rates. The findings suggest that, for Ashkenazi and Shepardic immigrant Jews, the environment modifies the difference in risk for developing MS determined by their genetic heritage. Thus, Israeli migration studies suggest that environmental factors might alter (increase or decrease) the inherited risks of MS that are associated with someone's racial ancestry.

Another type of epidemiological study that bolsters arguments for some environmental factor involves exploring so-called epidemics of MS—instances where many more cases of MS occur than would be expected based on geographic location and characteristics of the local population. One MS epidemic that attracted considerable interest involves the isolated Faroe Islands, a semi-independent territory of Denmark between Iceland and Norway and originally settled by the Norse Vikings, with a population in 1998 of approximately 44,000 inhabitants (Kurtzke, 2000). Before July 1943, no Faroese were known to have had MS according to records dating back to 1900. However, within two years of the April 1940 arrival of British troops stationed on the Faroe Islands during World War II, native-born Faroese began being diagnosed with MS. In the first wave of the epidemic, from 1941 to 1944, 21 Faroese developed MS. For five years during World War II, up to 7,000 military personnel from Great Britain encamped near Faroese villages across the islands, and growing numbers of natives developed the disease.

Researchers drew maps, carefully noting British troop locations on the Faroe Islands and pinpointing the location and the timing of the newly diagnosed MS cases. These maps showed close proximity between the British camps and new MS cases. In addition, at least two years needed to elapse between the arrival of the British and the diagnosis of MS among their Faroese neighbors. Kurtzke (2000) speculated that the best explanation for this geographic clustering and the delayed timing of MS diagnoses among the Faroese is an infection carried by the troops: specifically, an infection affecting a large proportion of the British military personnel but not causing infectious symptoms (since these were healthy troops); and a two-or-more-year lag before symptoms of MS appear. In other words, at least a two-year incubation period must elapse between exposure to the infection from the British troops and development of MS among the native Faroese. Various researchers have explored different possible infectious agents, including the possibility of canine distemper. Perhaps the dogs that accompanied British troops carried the offending virus.

Despite these and other interesting observations from epidemiologic studies, little is known about precisely what environmental factors might be responsible for altering the risks of developing MS. Scientists have invested considerable effort in trying to identify specific environmental triggers without conclusive success. Currently, environmental contributors to MS remain enigmatic—strongly presumed but not yet proven.

Studies have explored whether viral illnesses in childhood might be linked to the subsequent development of MS. Researchers have examined the blood of persons with and without MS looking for evidence (antibody titers) of exposure to certain viruses. Some studies have considered viruses that cause the common childhood infections of measles, mumps, and rubella; none have found associations with MS. Other research has explored possible roles for such viruses as rabies, herpes simplex viridae, parainfluenza 1, and human retroviruses. It seems that, every few years, a new virus or infectious agent attracts active investigation, only to yield no connection between the virus and MS.

One virus that has attracted more attention is the Epstein-Barr virus (EBV), a herpesvirus (*Human herpesvirus 4*) that causes infectious mononucleosis. (The virus was named after British virologists Michael A. Epstein and Yvonne M. Barr, who first isolated the virus in 1964. In addition to mononucleosis, the Epstein-Barr virus is associated with a cancer called Burkitt's lymphoma.) Studies have found higher rates of MS among persons with evidence of EBV exposure, especially those who had infectious mononucleosis at relatively young ages (less than 18 years of age). The fact that EBV exposure is so common in the population complicates efforts to implicate EBV in development of MS. Nonetheless, other studies have suggested that there may be some linkage between the body's response to EBV and development of autoimmune diseases.

While no final conclusions regarding the role of EBV and MS have been reached, this area remains under investigation. Some experts are wary about assigning a role to EBV for the development of MS. In contrast, others assert that EBV infection is a strong risk factor for MS but that EBV alone cannot explain fully the epidemiology of MS. These experts suggest that EBV likely interacts with some other factor, either infectious or noninfectious, to cause MS.

SUNLIGHT EXPOSURE, VITAMIN D, AND MS

Given the relationship between latitude and MS prevalence, some researchers have turned to perhaps the most obvious explanation: intensity of sun exposure (Ascherio and Munger, 2008). Might longer hours and greater intensity of solar radiation protect persons living closer to the equator from developing MS? Could childhood exposures to sunlight also affect the likelihood of MS developing during adult years?

Scientists are considering several possibilities for a potential role of sunlight exposure. Ultraviolet (UV) radiation from sunlight can suppress the immune system, which in turn might lower risks of MS. Another possibility involves vitamin D (nicknamed the sunshine vitamin)—a vitamin naturally produced when the human body is exposed to sunlight. Specifically, ultraviolet B (UVB) radiation in sunlight prompts 7-dehydrocholesterol in human skin to convert to previtamin D_3, which then undergoes a series of transformations resulting finally in biologically active vitamin D.

At latitudes greater than 42°—the latitude of Boston, Massachusetts, for example—UVB radiation is absorbed by the atmosphere in the winter, so that vitamin D levels fall even among persons who are frequently outdoors and exposed to sunlight during winter months. Blood tests show that average vitamin D levels have a strong latitude gradient, declining with increasing distance from the equator. Persons can consume vitamin D in their diets. Vitamin D is plentiful in such foods as fish and liver oils, egg yolks, and vitamin D–fortified milk.

One hypothesis undergoing active investigation is whether vitamin D deficiencies (low levels of vitamin D) increase the risk of developing MS. Conversely, higher levels of vitamin D could protect against the disease. These possibilities could explain the latitude gradient of MS (see Figure 3.1), as well as findings from migration studies, if childhood sun exposures and thus natural vitamin D production determine adult risks. Many, although not all, epidemiological studies lend support to the possibilities that vitamin D might reduce the risk of developing MS and that vitamin D levels during childhood and early adolescence are critically important. Scientists in the laboratory are exploring ways that vitamin D might prevent autoimmune diseases, including MS. Vitamin D could possibly affect regulatory T cells (see Chapter 4), but more research is needed to understand these effects.

If vitamin D reduces the risk of developing MS, some advocate giving supplements to boost vitamin D levels, especially in adolescents and young adults. Taking too much vitamin D, however, can cause complications, including nausea, vomiting, constipation, and weakness, among other problems. Excessive amounts of vitamin D can elevate the level of calcium in the blood, which can produce mental confusion and dangerous changes in heart rhythm. More research is needed to explore whether vitamin D supplements can help prevent MS and, if so, to determine appropriate daily vitamin D doses to achieve this benefit.

CIGARETTE SMOKING AND MS

Finally, epidemiological studies find that MS occurs at higher rates among tobacco smokers than nonsmokers (Ascherio and Munger, 2008, 25). Cigarette use does not explain the worldwide patterns of MS, and many with the disease (such as myself) have never smoked. But smoking is increasingly recognized as a potentially critical risk factor for the disease.

Studies have found that the risk of developing MS rises with increasing cigarette consumption and length of time persons have smoked. Heavy smokers are 70 percent more likely to develop MS than are nonsmokers. Other research suggests that MS disability progresses significantly faster among smokers compared with persons who have never smoked. Smokers with relapsing-remitting MS (see Table 2.1) advance to secondary progressive MS much more quickly than do nonsmokers.

Researchers are trying to understand exactly how cigarette smoking might increase risks of MS. The observation that smokers are also more likely to contract other autoimmune diseases, such as rheumatoid arthritis, raises questions about whether smoking affects the body's immune system. Another possibility involves effects of nicotine or nitrous oxide from cigarette smoke on the brain.

These observations underscore the urgency of encouraging persons with MS who smoke to quit and those who do not smoke to avoid cigarettes. Persons with a close relative with MS should be especially warned against cigarette smoking, since their risks are already higher because of genetic factors. One estimate suggests that eliminating smoking could prevent up to 6 percent of MS cases in the United States.

CONCLUSIONS

Epidemiological studies of MS reach back to shortly after Charcot first systematically described the disease. Despite 150 years of tracking MS in populations around the globe, epidemiological researchers have provided few definitive answers about what causes MS. Building upon studies of relatives of persons with MS, scientists have identified clues about the contribution of genetics. While the worldwide population distribution of MS offers tantalizing hints of environmental causes, efforts to disentangle the evidence have not produced definitive answers about environmental links. Recent studies about sunlight exposure and a potentially protective role of vitamin D are intriguing. But future research will need to determine whether vitamin D supplements, particularly in youth and early adulthood, could help prevent MS. Epidemiologic studies do provide good evidence that smoking increases the likelihood of MS, adding to the many other compelling health reasons to avoid cigarettes.

4

Role of the Immune System in Causing MS

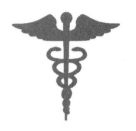

More than 20 years have elapsed since Sally Ann Jones's diagnosis (see Chapter 2). During that time, MS has limited her mobility and caused many other physical difficulties. But, she says, "I'm never sick—not with anything other than MS stuff." She rarely gets the common contagious viral infections, such as the colds that cause short-term misery for millions of persons every year. Mrs. Jones has thought deeply about this and has an explanation: "I guess my immune system is always working. It's always turned on fighting every little thing."

Mrs. Jones might be correct—perhaps her immune system is hypervigilant, constantly on the lookout for potential infectious threats. That hyperactive state could offer some benefits. Common viral infections might occur 20 percent to 50 percent less often in persons with MS than among similar persons who do not have MS (Sibley, Bamford, and Clark, 1985). Possibly persons with MS have better immune system defenses against common viruses than do other individuals. However, a countervailing downside might swamp this small benefit. MS relapses seem to occur at two to three times higher rates during periods immediately following common viral infections than at other times. Perhaps when persons with MS do succumb to common viral illnesses, their immune systems go into hyperdrive, with negative consequences for their MS.

As described in earlier chapters, since Charcot first recognized MS as a specific disease in the mid-nineteenth century, physicians and neuroscientists have generated numerous theories about its cause. Infections, toxic exposures, genetics, and other possible causes have dominated speculation over the last 150 years. Although research findings from the 1930s raised questions about a potential role for immune mechanisms (biological processes related to immune system functions), only in the 1960s did scientists begin seriously to consider this possibility. Starting in the 1970s, most research on causes of MS has investigated immune mechanisms, and researchers have published more than 7,000 scientific articles in medical journals on this topic. Since the 1980s, efforts to treat MS have focused primarily on modifying patients' immune systems or immunological responses (see Chapter 7).

This chapter examines the possible role of the immune system in causing MS, exploring evidence that supports this theory and how immune mechanisms might work. The chapter starts by briefly introducing how the human immune system functions and then discusses special features relating to immunological activities in the central nervous system (behind the so-called blood-brain barrier). Although today many scientists believe that autoimmune processes—where the body's immune system attacks its own tissues or cells—cause MS plaques, not everyone agrees. Even if autoimmune processes do cause MS plaques, this fact does not address the more fundamental question of what stimulates the body's immune system to behave in such a self-destructive fashion. Furthermore, autoimmune attacks do not explain the degeneration of neuronal axons, which is a key pathological feature of MS. Thus, much remains unclear about the role of the immune system in MS.

OVERVIEW OF THE IMMUNE SYSTEM

As described by the National Institute of Allergy and Infectious Diseases (NIAID, 2007), the immune system is a complex network involving millions of cells, tissues, and organs working together as the body's front line of defense against foreign substances, bacteria, viruses, parasites, and other microscopic invaders. An effective defense requires that the immune system perform three basic functions. First, it must recognize an invader (such as a virus or substance) as foreign and threatening, something to expel from the body. Second, once the immune system identifies a foreign threat, it must mobilize its forces to combat the invader. Finally, the immune system must recognize when it has succeeded in destroying the threat, call off its mobilized defense team, and clean up the microscopic debris left behind by the battle, making the site of invasion as healthy as possible so that normal functioning can resume.

The first step—recognizing an invader as foreign—seems straightforward. However, performing this task is extraordinarily complex. The cells at the front lines of the immune system must have some way to distinguish self (the body's own cells and substances) from foreign invaders, the nonself. To allow this to happen, all cells have surface marker molecules, which are genetically determined and unique to each individual (identical twins are the exception, with identical marker molecules because they have identical genes). When immune system cells encounter other cells with these self-marker molecules, they normally coexist without attacking. Anything that is recognized as foreign or nonself and therefore triggers an immune response is called an antigen.

The second step in the immune system response is mobilizing to destroy the foreign invader. Various players in the immune response interact within a complex network, called synonymously the lymph, lymphoid, or lymphatic system. Much of the lymphatic system parallels the circulatory system of arteries, capillaries, and veins through which blood travels to and from all parts of the body. The primary organs of the lymphatic system are the following:

- Bone marrow, the soft tissue filling the hollow cores of bones, where all blood cells originate (including red blood cells, which transport oxygen, and white blood cells, including lymphocytes and other inflammatory cells, which conduct the immune response);
- Thymus, a butterfly-shaped organ located at the base of the neck behind the sternum or breastbone, where certain types of immune cells mature;
- Spleen, a flat curved organ located in the left side of the abdomen under the diaphragm (opposite the liver, which is underneath the diaphragm on the right), which has several functions, including filtering and storing blood, harboring immune system cells, and serving as the staging area for immune cells to confront antigens; and
- Lymph nodes, small bean-shaped structures congregating at various positions strategically placed around the body (such as in the neck, the armpits, and groin), which filter lymphatic fluids and also host attacks of immune cells on antigens.

Lymphatic vessels connect these organs. These delicate microscopic vessels, often channeled alongside arteries, veins, and capillaries, transport lymph, a clear fluid that bathes tissues and also carries away the toxins and detritus produced as by-products of inflammatory immunologic attacks against foreign invaders. Thus, a major function of circulating lymph is to wash away the floating molecular equivalent of garbage and to keep bodily tissues pristine and healthy.

Two primary types of cells, collectively called lymphocytes (cyte means cell), conduct the immune response: T lymphocytes (or simply T cells), named T after the thymus where they mature after leaving the bone marrow; and B lymphocytes (B cells). When triggered by an antigen, B cells mature into their activated form called plasma cells, which produce antibodies customized to bind with specific antigens. Also called immunoglobulins, antibodies are large protein molecules, typically comprised of four subunits, two light chains (short segments of protein) and two heavy chains (longer protein segments). Antibodies coat enemy cells or substances floating in the bloodstream or lymph. These antibodies signal to other immune system cells that an invader is present, triggering a destructive inflammatory response by recruiting various white blood cells to the enemy's location. Millions of different B cells are preprogrammed to produce antibodies against millions of very specific antigens, such as the virus causing common colds or the pneumococcus bacterium causing pneumonia. B cells do not themselves attack enemy cells or substances.

T cells come in two major subtypes, which play very different roles. First, regulatory or helper T cells (also called Th cells) function as their name suggests, by communicating with other cells and coordinating the immune response. Through their chemical messages, Th cells orchestrate various actions, such as stimulating B cells nearby to make antibodies, activating other T cells, or telling activated cells to stand down once the enemy is vanquished.

Second, cytotoxic T lymphocytes, also called killer T cells, can directly attack and destroy invading cells. Killer T cells must recognize invaders that carry nonself molecular markers on their surface and distinguish enemies from self, which should not be destroyed. Killer T cells can bind to the nonself invaders and destroy them with lethal chemicals called cytokines.

Unlike B cells, T cells do not recognize and react to antigens floating in their local environments. Instead, T cells circulate widely throughout the body, patrolling constantly for foreign invaders. They respond to antigens only when specific marker molecules recognized as self present the antigen to the T cell. These self marker molecules on cells are genetically encoded on a section of chromosome 6 called the major histocompatibility complex (MHC), mentioned in Chapter 3 (section on genetics and MS). In humans, these MHC encoded marker molecules are called human leukocyte antigens (HLAs).

Almost every cell in the body has MHC marker molecules covering its surface, which allow T cells to distinguish self from nonself. In addition, MHC-determined molecules present foreign antigens to killer T cells. If a killer T cell recognizes a nonself MCH marker molecule or antigen on the surface of a nearby cell, it will destroy that nonself cell by binding to the cell and injecting it with deadly cytokines.

BLOOD-BRAIN BARRIER

The immune system uses elaborate processes to send messages throughout the body, calling immune cells to congregate at locations where a nonself threat exists and also dispersing gathered cells once the threat is extinguished. In particular, chemical signals called lymphokines summon activated killer T cells to particular sites where they must destroy enemy invaders. Following a lymphokine alert, for example, activated killer T cells will track down and attack cells infected with viruses. In order to enter the tissues and battle the enemy invader, these activated cells must pass through the wall (which is called the endothelium) of the vessel through which they traveled to the location. Various chemicals released by activated cells relax endothelial barriers, allowing the cells to transmigrate or translocate across the vessel wall into the tissues to perform their mission.

The process of releasing lymphokines in the circulating bloodstream and deploying chemicals that permit cells to migrate across endothelial vessel walls works efficiently throughout the body, sending activated immune cells to microscopic battlefields. But, as described in Chapter 1, the central nervous system is special. It is guarded not only by bony structures and multiple layers of tissues but also by the protective blood-brain barrier—specialized properties of the microscopic blood vessels and their endothelial walls that prevent certain molecules and activated cells from passing into central nervous system tissues. The blood-brain barrier presents the final impediment that cells and molecules must traverse to enter the tightly shielded sanctuary of the central nervous system. This microscopic barrier is remarkably effective at keeping potentially damaging cells and chemicals from invading the central nervous system.

While tiny molecules such as oxygen, carbon dioxide, and ethanol can diffuse easily across the endothelial walls of central nervous system capillaries, many other molecules cannot, halted by the blood-brain barrier. Passage of cells and larger molecules across this endothelial barrier requires various complicated processes, involving complex carrier mechanisms and transport molecules. If the transport processes do not function or permit passage, these molecules and cells cannot penetrate into brain and spinal cord tissues. To treat tumors in the brain with particular chemotherapy drugs, for instance, cancer doctors must inject these medications directly into the CSF using a lumbar puncture: the drugs will not pass through the blood-brain barrier to reach the brain tumor if they are infused into the bloodstream via an arm vein. Similarly, except in specific circumstances, the blood-brain barrier typically keeps activated lymphocytes out of central nervous system tissues.

AUTOIMMUNE DISORDERS AND MS

In MS, two aspects of the immune system appear to malfunction, resulting in an inflammatory immune response that damages the body's own tissues (see Figure 4.1). First, immune system cells attack and destroy the myelin sheaths encasing neuronal axons and possibly the oligodendrocytes that produce these laminar myelin structures (Chapter 1). Second, the blood-brain barrier relaxes, allowing activated T cells, other inflammatory cells, and molecules (such as certain lymphokines) that should ordinarily remain outside the central nervous system to enter its precincts. Activated and directed by the lymphokines, migrating T cells join the B lymphocytes normally residing within the central nervous system and other inflammatory cells in attacking myelin sheaths and their associated oligodendrocytes.

When a body's immune system attacks its own tissues, erroneously treating them as nonself, this is called an autoimmune response or process. Autoimmune processes cause a variety of diseases affecting different parts of the body. For example, some types of diabetes and arthritis are autoimmune disorders, where the body's immune system attacks its own tissues: cells in the pancreas that produce insulin for Type I diabetes, and joints for rheumatoid and certain other forms of arthritis.

Many experts believe MS is an autoimmune disease, in which the immune system mistakenly destroys or damages the myelin sheaths surrounding neural axons and possibly their associated oligodendrocytes (NINDS, 2009). Exactly how such damage and cell death occurs remains unclear, although several simultaneous processes likely contribute to the destruction. Killer T cells may injure

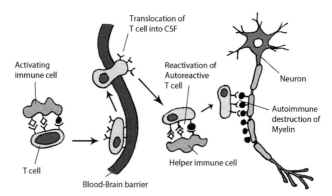

Figure 4.1. Autoimmune Attack on Myelin Sheaths. This schematic shows how activated T cells might pass across the blood-brain barrier into the central nervous system to destroy the myelin sheaths surrounding the axons of neurons. [Anil Shukla]

the myelin sheaths, along with their oligodendrocytes, by erroneously recognizing them as nonself, binding onto them, and injecting them with lethal lymphokine chemicals. Helper T cells might mediate this destruction by secreting substances that summon and activate other inflammatory cells such as macrophages, a specific type of immune system cell that destroys and consumes foreign invaders. Under the microscope, most, although not all, myelin sheaths undergoing active destruction are swarming with inflammatory cells—especially helper T cells releasing substances that orchestrate the immune response—congregating around the blood vessels that supply surrounding tissues.

Researchers speculate that a particular component of myelin called myelin basic protein serves as the antigen that stimulates the autoimmune response. They base this speculation largely on studies in which laboratory animals receive injections of myelin basic protein and develop a condition (experimental allergic encephalomyelitis) that closely resembles MS. In these animal studies, the injected myelin basic protein appears to stimulate activation of antimyelin killer T cells, which then attack the animal's own myelin sheaths.

Scientists have also explored how abnormal relaxation of blood-brain barrier defenses allows activated T cells and immune system substances to enter the central nervous system (Bar-Or, 2006). Several processes seem to contribute to the breakdown of the blood-brain barrier, including an enzyme that disrupts the matrix material holding together the vascular wall or endothelium. Activated T cells easily cross the blood-brain barrier because carrier mechanisms and transport molecules are upregulated, speeding their passage.

Other intriguing clues suggest immune system involvement in myelin destruction. As noted above, self marker molecules on cells are genetically encoded on the MHC section of chromosome 6; MHC encoded marker molecules in humans are called HLA. HLA patterns in persons with MS tend to differ from those of individuals without the disease. In particular, among white northern Europeans and Americans, certain HLA types (such as HLA-DR2) are much more common in persons with MS than in those without MS. Different HLA patterns correspond to variations in the course and severity of MS.

QUESTIONS ABOUT AUTOIMMUNE CAUSES

While many scientists believe that MS is an autoimmune disease, skeptics remain. Some role for the immune system seems obvious—the congregation of lymphocytes and other inflammatory cells at the site of myelin destruction is visible through the lens of the microscope. However, not all MS plaques demonstrate this cellular invasion: myelin destruction can occur without swarms of lymphocytes and macrophages. How and why these immune system cells arrive at the myelin plaques and what exactly they are doing there remains unclear. Furthermore, immune system cells appear at lesions in other neurological conditions, such as head injuries, strokes, and various neurodegenerative diseases.

The leading question about a potential autoimmune mechanism for MS is what exactly triggers the response: what causes the body's immune system to attack itself? Speculation focuses on environmental factors, such as the viruses mentioned in Chapter 3, with several possible explanations (Lipton et al., 2007). Constantly vigilant, the body's immune system sensing a viral incursion could activate an aggressive response to destroy the invader. Perhaps the body's immune system, mobilized to seek and eliminate the virus, makes a mistake known as molecular mimicry—where a molecular region on the surface of the virus tricks immune cells into destroying the body's own tissues that have similar surface markers.

Another possibility is that myelin damage occurs as a by-product of an exuberant attack against an actual virus in its midst. The chemicals and other substances released by immune cells combating a viral infection may produce collateral damage, injuring nearby tissues that were not the target of the attack. Under this scenario, the damage is not actually autoimmune but instead is analogous to injuring a bystander unlucky enough to live near a battlefield.

While earlier researchers focused on myelin damage as the initial injury within MS plaques, the possibility that oligodendrocyte death is the instigating event raises new speculation. Perhaps a persistent viral infection of oligodendrocytes could start the destructive immunological response. Myelin destruction and oligodendrocyte death could occur as the immune system repeatedly combats a tenacious viral invader embedded within these critical glial cells. Death of oligodendrocytes could precipitate several responses, including degeneration of the attached myelin sheath and activation of T and B lymphocytes. Macrophages could arrive to cleanse the site of myelin debris and eliminate remnants of cell destruction.

Finally, some researchers are troubled by the absence of inflammatory cells, including lymphocytes and macrophages, at the sites of perhaps one-third of MS plaques. Maybe the immune system plays no role in causing MS (Chaudhuri and Behan, 2004). Various alternative explanations involve metabolic mechanisms, such as effects of vitamin D and sunlight exposure as described in Chapter 3. Under these theories, metabolic abnormalities of neurons and supporting glial cells in the central nervous system cause disease progression and breakdown of the blood-brain barrier. These metabolic deficiencies lead ultimately to degeneration of neurons in the brain and spinal cord and thus impair their functioning.

Today, some experts argue that, over the lifetime, there are two pathological processes at play in MS. During autoimmune activity, myelin sheaths are attacked and destroyed. Under the microscope, these acute lesions are teaming with immune cells. However, this autoimmune activity is most active during early years of the disease. Also starting early—but continuing in later years of illness—the degenerative process destroys neuronal functioning. Degeneration involves the progressive deterioration of the cellular integrity of neurons and axons, with replacement by fibrosis or degraded cells that no longer function normally. Thus, over time, degeneration becomes the dominant pathological process in the central nervous system of persons with MS.

CHALLENGES AND IMPLICATIONS OF FINDING A CAUSE

The damage of MS occurs at the cellular or even molecular level in living, breathing people, in the most protected and functionally critical part of the body—the central nervous system. Unlike cancerous tumors elsewhere in the body, which can be spotted on X-ray and biopsied to extract malignant tissues for microscopic and biochemical analysis, it is impossible to detect, localize, and biopsy newly forming MS plaques. Someday, new imaging techniques may allow scientists to noninvasively examine the molecular biology of developing MS lesions. Today, however, the tools for understanding MS plaques, degenerative changes of neurons, and the underlying cause of MS are crude.

Some cellular or molecular causes might prove especially elusive to detect. Persistent virus infections are notoriously hard to find and prove, for a variety of reasons. Most obvious, obtaining tissue from the brain or spinal cord to perform rigorous viral studies is neither ethical nor practical. Taking tissues from critical central nervous system locations could leave a patient with permanent functional deficits. Technical problems, such as difficulties culturing viruses and absent markers of intracellular viral infestations, also impede detection of persistent viral infections.

While debates about the causes of MS might seem esoteric, they hold critical implications for treatments. As described in Chapter 6, major breakthroughs in MS treatment over the last two decades have assumed an immunological basis for the disease. Recent treatments have focused on specific aspects of immune system functioning. The fact that these new treatments often provide only minimal benefits—and offer no help at all to some patients—raises questions about whether these interventions are pursuing the correct target. Perhaps immune system dysfunctions do cause MS, but current therapies have not yet targeted the actual mechanism of disease. In particular, treatments have not yet figured out how to stop the degenerative processes that appear to dominate after initial immunological attacks. Reversing degeneration or restoring function to damaged cells is the next huge challenge for MS therapeutics.

5

Symptoms and Diagnosis of MS

As its name suggests, MS arrives in multiple guises and can take many different twists and turns over a patient's lifetime. Specific symptoms depend on what part of the brain or spinal cord the disease attacks. All persons with MS have their own unique stories. Some individuals have one or two mild flares of symptoms, develop few if any impairments, and are never definitively diagnosed. In contrast, others experience widely ranging symptoms that become profoundly disabling. While the vast majority of persons with MS have a fairly normal life expectancy, a small fraction of persons die within several years of diagnosis from rapidly progressive debility. The stories of Joni and Jenny exemplify this diversity.

Joni is in her mid-40s. She runs a small flower shop and has always been busy and physically active. For 20 years, she had periodically experienced sensory symptoms that were episodic (would come and go over weeks or months), such as numbness and tingling shifting around different parts of her legs, torso, and arms. Between these occasional episodes, she felt perfectly fine. Then, after those 20 years, Joni began having significant difficulty walking. Her legs felt heavy, like they were encased in concrete, making every movement an exhausting struggle. Joni visited a neurologist, who diagnosed MS based on her long history of waxing and waning symptoms. She is still walking slowly and arduously with a cane, but she worries about the future.

Jenny is in her early-40s. In high school, she was very athletic, playing soccer and running track. However, Jenny remembers always seeming to trip and fall, spraining her ankle, much more often than the other girls. She went to nursing school and after graduating started working in a hospital emergency room (ER). ER duty is physically demanding, with nurses continually on their feet and their minds constantly on alert, running urgently from one crisis to another over long hours. During these lengthy shifts, Jenny began noticing odd sensations. The first was something called Lhermitte's sign, a tingly electrical sensation tracking down the arms, back, or legs after flexing the neck or bowing one's head. (Lhermitte's sign also occurs in other conditions, such as after head or neck injuries, but it is often the first noticeable symptom of what is eventually diagnosed as MS. The sign was named after French neurologist Jacques Jean Lhermitte, who described it in a 1924 article, although it had been reported by other physicians in the 1910s.)

On busy days in the ER, Jenny developed difficulties doing tasks with her hands and fingers, such as inserting intravenous lines and drawing blood. But she kept on working, thinking maybe she was having problems with circulation in her fingertips. Then, Jenny began having trouble articulating words, and her speech sounded slightly slurred. She worried a little that people might think she was drunk, especially since her walking had become somewhat unsteady.

"On late nights in the ER, I'd just brush it away," Jenny recalled. "I kept on working, with symptoms coming and going for maybe a year or two. Then one hot July, things started getting really bad." Jenny's July troubles were not surprising. As described in Chapter 2, French neurologist Charles Prosper Ollivier d'Angers in the early 1800s had described the extraordinary heat sensitivity of many persons with MS. Jenny developed urinary incontinence (inability to hold her urine). With her walking troubles, Jenny fell and went to her own ER for evaluation of an ankle sprain.

> From that point on, I never really got back to where I was before. I started using a cane, and I had to stop working as an ER nurse. I began having flares every six months. I had all sorts of sensory problems—numbness, tingling. My speech was still slurry, and my walking went downhill with terrible spasms in my right leg that were hard to control. And I had troubles with double vision, although that fortunately got better.

Jenny started using a scooter-type wheelchair about five years later. Now she needs help doing basic activities, such as getting dressed and preparing meals.

* * * * *

MS varies along two primary dimensions—over time and across a range of symptoms. Since the disease is incurable, patients can experience a wide variety of symptoms, which, as for Jenny, begin to accumulate and become disabling over the years. Although each person's story is unique, MS follows four basic patterns in timing and extent of disability (see Table 2.1). This chapter describes these four patterns and reviews the range of symptoms common to MS, along with describing how neurologists assess patients for these different symptoms. Although sophisticated imaging scans and laboratory analyses might suggest a diagnosis of MS, the patient's clinical history—patterns of symptoms over time —remains the major factor in making the diagnosis.

PATTERNS OF MS

As mentioned in Chapters 2 and 3, the patterns of MS symptoms fall into four categories: relapsing-remitting, secondary progressive, primary progressive, and progressive relapsing (Olek, 2008c; NINDS, 2009).

About 85 percent of persons newly diagnosed with MS have the relapsing-remitting pattern of the disease. Relapsing-remitting MS usually appears between 15 and 50 years of age, occurring in two to three times more women than men. Joni's MS is a classic example of this common pattern. In the relapsing-remitting pattern, persons have relapses or flares of symptoms, which last for days, weeks, or months and then resolve (go away). Between these relapses, persons experience remissions where symptoms disappear for weeks or even years.

About 15 percent of persons with relapsing-remitting MS have a single flare and never have any other symptoms. Experts argue about what fraction of persons with lengthy remissions, during which they have no symptoms for 15 or more years, will go on to develop additional symptoms. Some unknown proportion of persons with relapsing-remitting disease may never be diagnosed with MS, if their symptoms are mild and periods of remission long. Studies of decedents (dead people) who have undergone autopsy have found significant numbers of brains and spinal cords with pathology suggestive of MS but no records that the persons while living reported MS-like symptoms or disability.

The majority of persons with relapsing-remitting MS go on to develop the second pattern of MS, the secondary progressive pattern: called secondary because it follows the initial relapsing-remitting presentation, and progressive because of accumulating disability. In secondary progressive MS, persons might continue to have flares, but their symptoms never completely resolve. Instead, difficulties persist, getting gradually worse with additional symptoms from new flares or exacerbations over time. Jenny's MS falls into this pattern. She started with problems "coming and going for maybe a year or two." Then, Jenny developed persistent symptoms, one after another, that never completely went away. Over time, the impairments accumulated, making Jenny unable to walk and needing assistance with basic daily activities.

The third pattern, primary progressive MS, occurs in about 10 percent of newly diagnosed individuals. It is typically identified at later ages than relapsing-remitting MS (between ages 30 and 60 years) and in equal numbers of men and women. As its name suggests, in primary progressive MS, persons experience a continual decline in functioning once disease symptoms start. They do not have the acute flares or attacks characteristic of relapsing-remitting MS, and their symptoms never resolve or disappear. Despite this, the progression of symptoms can be quite slow, although some persons experience rapid declines (becoming profoundly disabled in a few years). Persons with primary progressive MS generally have a worse prognosis or outlook for long-term disability than those who start with relapsing-remitting MS.

The fourth and rarest pattern is progressive relapsing MS, which has similar age and sex distributions as primary progressive MS and affects about 5 percent of patients. In this pattern, impairments progress from the onset of symptoms. But persons also have acute flares or relapses, with or without some degree of recovery, between these exacerbations.

In rare instances, MS occurs in children, defined here as persons younger than 16 years old. Pediatric MS (MS in children) might account for 5 percent of total cases of MS, but exact numbers remain unclear. As in adults, the course of pediatric MS is highly variable. The disease may progress more slowly in children than in adults. But because children are diagnosed at much younger ages, they might experience disability at earlier ages than persons diagnosed as adults.

Although this discussion draws clear distinctions between the four patterns of MS, for most patients with new symptoms of MS, their future disease course is uncertain. While the majority of persons with relapsing-remitting MS go on to develop secondary progressive MS, some do not. Therefore, most persons newly diagnosed with MS face considerable uncertainty: what course will their disease take? They may not know which pattern of MS they have until many years later.

INTRODUCTORY COMMENTS ABOUT MS SYMPTOMS

As described in Chapter 1, MS is a degenerative disease of the central nervous system (brain and spinal cord). Each section of the central nervous system performs specific functions. Figure 5.1 shows the so-called dermatomes—skin surfaces of the body controlled by each of the paired spinal nerves that emanate

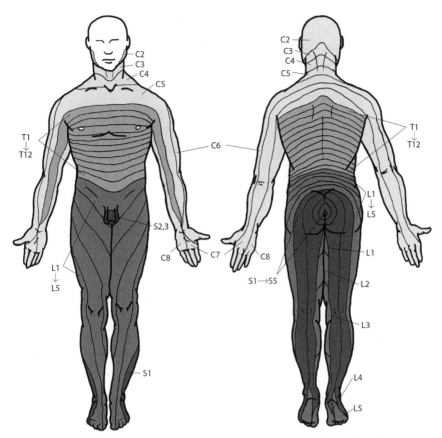

Figure 5.1. Dermatomes. This figure shows the dermatomes, which are the skin surfaces supplied by the spinal nerves. C = cervical, T = thoracic, L = lumbar, and S = sacral. T5 is the 5th thoracic spinal nerve, and so on. [Anil Shukla]

from the spinal cord—and Figure 5.2 shows a spinal cord cross-section (what one would see cutting across the spinal cord) that highlights various different nerve tracts. If lesions occur within a particular spinal nerve or tract within the spinal cord, the functions controlled by those regions will be impaired. Similarly, depending on the location of lesions within the brain itself, MS can impair or disturb a wide range of functions, from thinking complex thoughts to seeing to moving a specific muscle.

Before discussing the range of MS symptoms, it is important to underscore several points. Sometimes MS symptoms are subtle, hard to pick up without a skilled examiner to both elicit information from the patient and to perform a meticulous neurological examination. Since symptoms can come and go, as in

Sensory Tracts (afferent)   Motor Tracts (efferent)

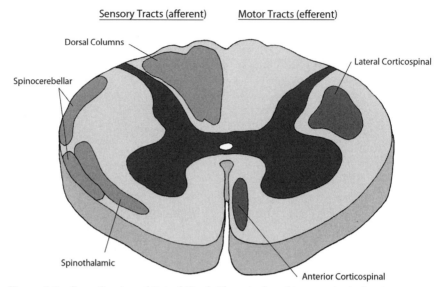

Figure 5.2. Cross-Section of Spinal Cord. The spinal cord is comprised of various tracts (or bundles) of nerves, which serve specific purposes. This schematic shows nerve tracts that convey sensory information from the body up to different parts of the brain (afferent sensory tracts) and tracts that send information from the brain down to muscles in the body (efferent). Many other tracts are not depicted in this simple drawing. [Anil Shukla]

relapsing-remitting MS, by the time the patient visits the neurologist, a specific problem may no longer exist or be easily detectable. Furthermore, because of their waxing and waning course and origins in the depths of the central nervous system, symptoms of MS can be very difficult for patients to describe in words. As patients start to compose verbal descriptions, they might pause, saying to themselves, "This sounds crazy. Who would believe me? People are going to think I am out of my mind." This fear of being disbelieved or ridiculed can cause patients to hesitate to tell others, even their doctors, about their sensations.

Here's an example of a bizarre symptom that is hard to describe in words, even for me—someone privileged with a medical degree and able to author this book! Sometimes, in the late afternoon when I am very tired—and especially when it is hot outside—I develop an uncomfortable sensation as if metal bands are encircling and constricting my torso, pressing in on my chest from all directions and making it feel hard for me to breathe in and out. Of course, there are no metal bands, and I am breathing perfectly normally, at a regular rate and rhythm. Very likely, this unnerving sensation relates to a lesion in the sensory tract of my spinal cord controlling my torso region. Although difficult to describe and comprehend, this recurrent and unpleasant sensation is nevertheless intensely real to me.

Several years ago, when interviewing other people with MS for a research project, some persons mentioned virtually this same symptom. They used almost identical language as mine, such as "bands wrapped around and pressing on my chest." These interviewees came from different walks of life than I do. Nonetheless, we felt a common and validating bond, born not simply of shared experiences but equally importantly shared language and metaphor. We understood each other perfectly.

Needless to say, recognizing and describing the symptoms of MS, especially multiple symptoms that come and go, could become a full-time job. Persons with diverse symptoms could find themselves consumed by tracking every nuance and subtle shift in sensations. Some persons become absorbed with monitoring their MS symptoms. Others of us feel that we would get nothing else done if we concentrated solely on tracking our MS symptoms. Occasionally, symptoms demand immediate attention. Particularly challenging is deciding when some new symptom represents the start of a flare that needs neurological evaluation and possibly treatment. Over decades of living with MS, each of us finds our own strategy for dealing with these complexities.

SYMPTOMS OF MS

No symptoms are unique to MS: each can occur in a number of other neurological or medical conditions. Certain symptoms, however, occur frequently in persons with MS. Furthermore, a relapsing and remitting time course of these symptoms strongly suggests the possibility of MS, especially when the patient is a young adult with a history of other symptoms over time. Table 5.1 shows how often persons with MS who responded to the Sonya Slifka survey (see the description of the Sonya Slifka study in Chapter 3) reported experiencing different symptoms at the time of their interview. Fatigue was the most common problem, followed by walking difficulties and stiffness and spasms. The discussion below describes frequent symptoms of MS (McDonald and Compston, 2005; Olek, 2008a).

Abnormal Sensation

Virtually every person with MS experiences some sort of sensory symptoms at some point. Abnormal sensations in the legs or arms are the presenting (initial) symptoms in just over 30 percent of MS cases. Sensory symptoms generally result from lesions in various sensory tracts of the spinal cord, such as those relating to perceptions of temperature, vibration, pain, and light touch. Persons commonly describe these distorted sensations as numbness, tingling, tightness (such as the

Table 5.1
Current Symptoms of MS

Symptom	Percent[a]
Fatigue	83%
Difficulty walking	67
Stiffness and spasms	63
Bladder problems	60
Memory or other cognitive problems	56
Pain and other unpleasant sensations	54
Emotional or mood problems	38
Vision problems	37
Dizziness or vertigo	36
Bowel problems	35
Tremors	30
Sexual problems	30
Difficulty moving arms	24
Swallowing problems	22
Speech problems	20
Seizures	2

[a]Among the survey respondents, 14% had had MS for 5 years or less, and 33% had had MS for more than 20 years.
Adapted from Minden et al., 2006.

metaphorical bands constricting the chest mentioned above), extreme heat or extreme cold, and pins and needles. An intense itchy sensation, particularly on one side of the head or neck, is also common. Being overheated and fatigued can worsen these aberrant sensations. While patients may not necessarily describe the distorted sensations as explicitly painful, they can be intensely uncomfortable and thus cause considerable distress.

By knowing which spinal nerves and nerve tracts supply various parts of the body (see Figures 5.1 and 5.2), skilled neurologists can conduct physical examinations that isolate the likely area of the spinal cord affected by MS. To test the sensory pathways involving the spinal cord, neurologists often use very basic tools, such as a tuning fork (vibration sense), the fluffed tip of a cotton swab (light touch), and a lightly applied tip of a pin (sharp touch). By touching portions of the limbs and trunk systematically with these tools and asking patients to report their sensations, neurologists can map areas with abnormal sensation and then relate these regions back to spinal cord locations. This process can be intensely uncomfortable. Some patients experience an extreme pain radiating or rippling outward from the point of even the lightest pinprick, while others describe a light pinprick as an electric shock.

Additional sensory tracts in the central nervous system that are commonly affected involve the ability to feel vibrations or discern the position of a body part—all activities that are completely unconscious in persons without MS but contribute significantly to impaired functioning in persons with the disease. For example, unless the conscious mind knows the location of the fingers, it would be impossible to perform an intentional task (such as turning a page or writing one's name) with the hands. Neurologists test vibratory and position sense using very simple approaches. After rapping a tuning fork to start its vibration, the neurologist holds the stem of the tuning fork against the patient's great toe, for example, asking the patient to indicate when all vibrations stop. Patients with impaired vibration sense will say the tuning fork has stopped vibrating before these fine motions actually cease.

Testing position sense is equally simple. The neurologist asks the patient to close his or her eyes and then takes the patient's hand (or foot) and moves a digit (finger or toe) very slightly up or down. The neurologist tells the patient to indicate the direction of this tiny movement—up or down. Patients with impaired position sense cannot tell accurately (or easily) whether the neurologist moved their finger (or toe) up or down.

Sensory problems relating to the trigeminal nerve—also known as the fifth cranial nerve, which serves the face and jaw—are common in MS. Acute paroxysmal pain in facial muscles caused by trigeminal neuralgia can result, as can waves of spasms and twitching of facial muscles. While other conditions can cause trigeminal neuralgia, its occurrence in young adults raises questions about MS.

The Lhermitte's sign that Jenny described is another sensory symptom that portends MS. Lhermitte's sign occurs when individuals flex their necks or bow their heads, producing rapid waves of electrical or tingling sensations tracking down the arms, back, or legs. Tumors, problems involving the discs between the cervical vertebrae (such as herniation), injuries, and other abnormalities can also cause Lhermitte's phenomenon. But as with Jenny, this sign is the first sensory disturbance of MS in about 2 percent of patients.

Vision Problems

After sensory abnormalities, vision problems are the second most common presenting symptom of MS, occurring in about 16 percent of cases. The optic nerve, also known as the second cranial nerve, conducts visual information from the surface of the retina in the eye to the brain. Optic neuritis, or inflammation of the optic nerve, is the most common eye problem in MS. For patients, optic neuritis often starts with pain in one eye, which gets worse with movement of that eye. Vision loss follows the eye pain. Generally, the loss involves spots or missing areas within the visual field (entire expanse of space visible up, down, right, and left without moving the eye). In typical optic neuritis, losses are concentrated in the central portion of the visual field. Optic neuritis in persons with MS generally involves only one eye. If two eyes are affected, one eye is usually worse than the other. When persons do have problems affecting both eyes, some other cause is likely (such as a brain tumor pressing on the optic nerve).

Ophthalmologists can diagnose optic neuritis by performing careful examinations of patients' visual fields and vision within the visual field. They then use bright lights and magnifying lenses, looking through a dilated pupil, to examine the retina (sensory membrane, comprised of rods and cones, lining the posterior portion of the eye). Rods and cones in the retina take visual information conveyed through the lens of the eye and translate it into chemical signals, which then reach the brain through the optic nerve, thus producing visual images. Generally, the retina of someone who has had optic neuritis is paler in color than the retina of someone who has never had this optic nerve inflammation.

Within two to six months after an acute episode of optic neuritis, 90 percent of persons with MS regain normal vision. However, after recovering their vision, many persons with MS report that bright colors, especially red, no longer seem as bright or intense (colors are desaturated). Others describe a general sense that their vision is dimmer than it was previously.

Weakness and Other Motor Symptoms

Motor functioning refers to movement of muscles. Acute and subacute motor problems are the presenting symptoms of approximately 14 percent of MS cases. Areas in both the cerebral cortex of the brain and the spinal cord initiate, coordinate, and control the transmission of neuronal impulses governing motor functioning. MS lesions in any of these areas can cause a variety of motor symptoms, which in more advanced stages will require persons with MS to use wheelchairs and make other accommodations to meet their mobility needs.

Weakness is more common in the legs than the arms, due to MS lesions occurring more frequently in spinal cord motor tracts governing leg functioning. Eventually, muscles, especially in the lower legs, shrink in size as they weaken and persons are no longer physically vigorous and active. Another frequent motor problem involves spasticity: spasms or involuntary contractions of the muscles or muscle fibers, most common in the legs and sometimes the trunk and arms. Various simple actions can trigger these spasms, such as persons trying to stand up. An additional motor problem is clonus, when complex groups of muscles involuntarily contract and then partially relax, perhaps because of abnormal firing of motor neurons. When this process occurs recurrently (over and over again), clonus results, with its characteristic beating or pulsing repeated movements.

Neurologists test motor functioning in various ways, such as by simply watching patients (who can reasonably safely do so) walk. In addition, skilled neurologists know how strong normal arm and leg muscles are when patients perform certain actions, such as flexing their arm or lifting their thigh and keeping it elevated while seated. To test muscle strength, neurologists ask patients to perform simple actions, such as flexing their arm at the elbow and holding it flexed in place. Then the neurologist exerts a counter force: pulling the patient's forearm forward and trying to straighten the elbow and unbend the flexion against the patient's resistance. Neurologists judge the patient's strength based on the relative amount of effort the neurologist must expend to counteract the patient's muscle force. Testing of motor functioning can sometimes seem like a friendly tussling match between neurologists and patients.

Another physical examination maneuver involves testing for abnormal tendon reflexes. The most common tendon reflex test involves lightly tapping on the area just below the patella or knee cap with a hard rubber hammer. For persons with normal neurological functioning, the knee jerk reflex involves the lower leg slightly kicking outward gently after the hammer taps on the tendon. Persons with MS, however, can have exaggerated knee jerk reflexes, where the lower leg kicks out rapidly after even a minimal hammer tap. Sometimes, tests of tendon reflexes in the knee and other locations (such as ankle and elbow) can result in clonus, the sustained pulsing or beating movements described above.

Finally, as described in Chapter 2, a physical examination approach developed by Parisian physician Joseph-François-Félix Babinski in the late 1800s remains a mainstay of MS evaluations. The so-called Babinski reflex occurs when neurologists stimulate the outer or lateral part of the sole of the foot (such as by stroking or drawing a blunt, narrow instrument along its length). The toes of normal individuals curl under, while the great toe of many persons with MS flexes upward and other toes fan outward.

Coordination Problems and Ataxia

Abnormalities in the cerebellum of the brain and other central nervous system tracts can disrupt coordination with consequences ranging from slurred speech to imbalanced gait. This lack of coordination is called ataxia. Physicians assess coordination by asking persons to walk and watching for careening or imbalanced movements—so-called ataxic gait. Listening to patients' speech patterns could also identify coordination deficits. Coordination problems with the fingers and hands cause difficulties performing tasks requiring fine motor movements. Neurologists typically give patients simple tasks to assess coordination, such as asking patients to place one hand lightly on their knee and then flip the hand from palm up to palm down repeatedly, as quickly as they can. Persons with impaired coordination are unable to flip their hand's orientation rapidly, instead performing this simple task slowly and clumsily.

Another indication of abnormal coordination is an intention tremor— trembling or shaking movements that occur as persons try to perform a task. (This differs from tremors some people have at rest.) The finger-to-nose test elicits intention tremors in persons with this impairment. While patients are seated on an examining table facing the neurologist, the neurologist asks patients to touch their own noses with their index finger and then, as quickly as possible, touch the neurologist's finger, which the neurologist holds 12 to 18 inches from the patient's face. Patients must repeatedly touch their own noses and then the neurologist's finger, while the neurologist moves his or her finger unpredictably right, left, up, or down. Patients with coordination problems have difficulty with this task, with their hands and forearms wavering or trembling as they seek to touch their neurologist's finger.

Bladder and Bowel Problems

Problems with bladder and bowel functioning are common among persons with MS. As shown in Table 5.1, 60 percent of persons with MS report currently having bladder problems, and 35 percent report bowel difficulties. The extent of patients' bladder and bowel dysfunction often seems commensurate with the degree of difficulties with motor functioning. Urinary problems likely result from MS lesions involving the sacral region of the spinal cord (see Chapter 1).

In persons without neurological diseases, the urinary bladder is a fairly muscular organ, which during voiding contracts and squeezes out virtually all accumulated urine produced by the kidneys. Over time, the bladders of persons with MS can lose their muscular tone, becoming dilated and flaccid, unable to contract effectively to void all urine. Even after urinating, substantial pools of urine might remain in the bladder, without patients being aware of the residual urine because of defective sensory input from the bladder. Sometimes bladders that accumulate large quantities of urine can overflow, producing incontinence. Depending on the specific nature of the bladder problems, some MS patients must catheterize themselves: insert a narrow, sterile, plastic tube or catheter through their urethra into their bladder, allowing urine to drain through the tube by gravity. Others use devices or surgical diversions to continuously drain urine from the bladder

The most common urinary symptom is urgency: sudden and pressing sensations of needing to urinate and being unable to keep the urethral sphincter closed and thus prevent incontinence. When a bathroom is not nearby, urgency frequently does lead to urinary incontinence, with persons spilling their urine. Medications help some, but not all persons control their urine flow. Otherwise, persons accommodate the possibility of incontinence by wearing sanitary pads similar in design to those worn by women during periods of menstrual bleeding but made of specially absorbent material that soaks up and holds urine. It is important to diagnose the specific type of bladder problem to recommend the best treatment or accommodation.

Urologists—surgical specialists who are experts in urinary tract diseases—provide consultations concerning urinary problems to MS patients. Some academic medical centers have uroneurologists, subspecialized experts in neurological conditions affecting urinary tract function. Typically, evaluation of bladder function in patients with MS involves specialized diagnostic studies, such as ultrasound and other tests that measure voiding pressures and residual fluid volumes in the bladder.

In rare instances, bladder problems can cause difficulties upstream in the kidneys—vital organs essential for cleansing toxins from the body. For that reason, neurologists will often monitor kidney function in MS patients with significant bladder difficulties by doing blood tests measuring chemical markers (blood urea nitrogen, creatinine) that indicate kidney functioning. Urinary tract infections, which are especially common in women, can complicate MS-related bladder problems.

Bowel problems are also common in patients with MS, with constipation being the major difficulty. Constipation is especially problematic for persons with very limited mobility. Fecal incontinence can also occur, with patients unable to control anal sphincter functioning once the fecal expulsion process begins. Specific testing is not necessary to diagnose MS-related bowel problems: patients can give an effective history.

Although walking difficulties provide the iconic image of disability in MS—the young adult using a wheelchair—patients have told me that bladder and bowel incontinence is their most profoundly disabling symptom. Learning to use the toilet reliably and leaving diapers behind are among the major transitions of very early childhood, marking new self-awareness and self-control. To lose that control and risk the embarrassment of urine running down one's leg—or even worse, being unable to control passage of feces—can be an omnipresent and terrifying prospect. Persons may become unwilling to leave their homes without knowing whether they have convenient and accessible (configured for wheel-chair users) restroom options at their destination.

Despite this, few public discussions of the effects of MS focus on bladder and bowel incontinence—this topic represents a quintessential social taboo. Patients likewise will rarely raise a topic that can cause such embarrassment and shame, although, of course, incontinence is not their fault. Persons with MS can spend enormous effort and use considerable ingenuity to avoid the public humiliation of bladder or bowel incontinence. One woman put a makeshift toilet into her minivan, after affixing curtains to the windows.

Heat Sensitivity

As mentioned in Chapter 2, the French physician d'Angers observed that, when placed into a tub of hot water, some persons could not get out on their own. This hot bath test became an early staple of the diagnostic work-up for MS, but it was fortunately abandoned decades ago. With other diagnostic assessment approaches, neurologists no longer needed to challenge patients with immersions in hot water, which are meant to sap their strength and render them virtually helpless.

Small increases in body temperature significantly worsen the functioning of many, although not all, persons with MS. Functioning returns to baseline levels once the person cools off and has a chance to rest and recover from being overheated. The exact reason for this phenomenon is unclear, but experts suggest an analogous process to what happens when faulty electrical circuits overheat and malfunction. Demyelinated nerves, like poorly insulated electrical wiring, might become hypersensitive to heat, and conduction blockages might occur with increasing temperatures.

Patients can report heat hypersensitivity to their neurologists—no compelling clinical reason necessitates testing patients for this condition. Persons who are particularly sensitive to heat may need to avoid heat exposure whenever possible. Air conditioning during summer months and not going outside during scorching weather are obvious steps. Patients also might use cooler water when showering or bathing, and they should eschew hot tubs and steam baths.

Fatigue

Some persons with MS experience complete and overwhelming general fatigue, unrelated to their motor functioning or other MS symptoms or activity levels. Up to 80 percent of persons with MS will report such fatigue at some point, sufficiently profound that it interferes with their daily activities. Among the Sonya Slifka study participants, 83 percent reported fatigue (see Table 5.1). People can wake up exhausted, even if they feel they slept through the night. MS fatigue can be consuming, preventing persons from working and caring for themselves, their homes, and their families.

No objective test exists that measures the extent of MS fatigue. This can complicate a person's efforts to navigate the consequences of MS fatigue. Explaining overwhelming fatigue to family members, who themselves might feel stressed by an expanded burden of caregiving, can generate tensions and questions. Persons with MS fatigue may feel that others disbelieve their extreme exhaustion and view them as lazy or feigning debility. After all, they may look entirely well. Why are they so tired and unable to help out around the house or go to work?

Nonetheless, MS fatigue is very real, and neurologists have explored treatments for it (various drugs are now available, which can help some patients). However, before attributing exhaustion to MS fatigue, neurologists must rule out other potential causes. Especially among younger women, who are still actively menstruating and thus depleting bodily iron stores through blood loss every month, anemia is one possible cause of fatigue. Neurologists should evaluate patients for thyroid problems and depression, which can both produce profound fatigue.

Finally, other aspects of MS can disrupt sleep, thus causing or worsening fatigue. Spasticity of the legs, which results in thrashing in bed, can keep patients awake. Persons with limited bladder capacity, who must arise frequently to void during nighttime hours, might have problems entering the deep sleep cycles that provide refreshment and restorative rest. Patients should also be evaluated for other conditions that disturb sleep, such as sleep apnea.

Pain

More than 40 percent of persons with MS report some form of chronic pain sufficiently severe to diminish their quality of life. MS pain is often complex and difficult to describe. Unlike obvious causes of pain, such as a broken bone, MS pain originates deep within the central nervous system. Pain presents in MS with a wide variety of patterns and locations throughout the body. Sometimes the pain relates to sensory distortions, such as disordered temperature perceptions generating feelings of searing heat or burning sensations. Spasms or other involuntary muscle movements can produce pain. The trigeminal nerve dysfunction described above can cause excruciating facial pain. Back, joint, and other muscle pains can result from gait abnormalities. Persons can also experience sharp pains in their bowels or other internal organs. Depression can compound patients' perceptions of pain.

As in fatigue, no objective test can quantify and measure MS pain. Neurologists must therefore ask patients questions about pain and listen carefully as they describe their sensations. Sometimes patients do not use the words pain or painful to describe their unpleasant sensations, which seem distinct from the typical concept of pain (such as the broken bone). Instead patients might call these sensations unpleasant, uncomfortable, or use other more descriptive phrases. Treating MS pain remains perplexing and little studied, although some medications can ameliorate symptoms for certain patients. As a leading MS textbook notes, "Although interest in pain in multiple sclerosis has increased, . . . the topic is still unduly neglected" (McDonald and Compston, 2005, 316).

Vertigo and Hearing Problems

From 30 to 50 percent of persons with MS experience vertigo at some time. Vertigo is a sensation of imbalance or spinning in space, and it can severely disorient patients. For example, a patient lying in bed might feel that the room is careening around him or her, dipping and swirling. In its most extreme form, vertigo can cause vomiting, headache, and great difficulty walking, as patients feel they are gyrating and twisting in space. Vertigo is caused by lesions related to the eighth cranial nerve. Because of these origins, vertigo is often accompanied by symptoms of dysfunction in adjacent cranial nerves, such as double vision, facial numbness, and hearing symptoms.

While MS frequently affects vision (see the discussion of optic neuritis above), the consequences for hearing are more difficult to assess. MS can cause conditions called hyperacusis (hearing that is abnormally acute) and phonophobia (abnormal fear of sound). In these circumstances, patients experience certain sounds as painfully loud or uncomfortable to their ears and therefore try to avoid exposure to these noises. In relatively rare cases, persons can lose their hearing (become hard of hearing or even deaf). Sudden hearing loss generally occurs along with vertigo and other symptoms. In these rare instances, hearing loss generally affects only one ear, although bilateral deafness can occur. MS might also cause more subtle hearing loss, but this is a symptom that patients relatively seldom mention. Since other factors can cause hearing loss, such as exposure to high decibel noises at work and loud music through headphones, patients might attribute any diminution in hearing to other sources.

Sexual Dysfunction

Problems with sexual functioning are common among persons with MS, although they can originate from many different sources. Bladder or bowel incontinence, spasticity, and weakness can cause mechanical difficulties. Distorted sensations in the skin can make even tender and loving caresses feel uncomfortable and unwelcome. Without a partner who completely appreciates this dynamic, interpersonal relations can become strained, with the person with MS feeling physically distressed and poorly understood and the partner sensing rejection and withdrawal. Furthermore, the person with MS might feel embarrassed or unattractive because of various bodily changes wrought by the disease.

Beyond these causes, MS lesions involving various motor and sensory pathways can directly affect sexual functioning. From 40 to 50 percent of men can experience erectile dysfunction, to varying degrees. When attempting intercourse, they may have trouble achieving or maintaining an erection. Among women, loss of libido (sexual desire) is perhaps the most common problem, along with difficulties with vaginal lubrication and attaining orgasm. Some women, however, remain capable of orgasm, even when they have severely compromised bladder and bowel function.

Cognitive Problems

Cognitive activities include thinking, reasoning, remembering, finding words to convey thoughts, and imagining. From one-third to two-thirds of persons with MS experience some degree of cognitive difficulties. Cognitive problems result when the cerebral cortex of the brain is affected by MS lesions, with grey matter as well as white matter of the brain becoming atrophied or shrinking in size over time. Persons with the relapsing-remitting pattern of MS are less likely to experience cognitive difficulties than those with progressive patterns of disease.

Outright dementia, with severe memory loss and profound cognitive incapacity, is very unusual. The most common cognitive consequences include short-term memory loss, attenuated attention, decreased speed of processing information, and problems with abstract thinking. Sometimes these problems are subtle and not apparent to the patient. Neuropsychological testing can identify specific cognitive deficits. Importantly, depression can exacerbate cognitive problems or cause its own cognitive limitations, such as slowing thought processes, impairing concentration and attention, and compromising memory. Evaluating patients for depressive symptoms is thus critical when assessing potential cognitive dysfunction.

EFFECTS OF PREGNANCY ON MS

MS affects more women than men and typically strikes during childbearing years, raising the question of how pregnancy might affect the symptoms and progression or course of disease. Some studies suggest that women's symptoms improve during pregnancy and then worsen during the several months after giving birth. The temporary improvement while pregnant may relate to changes in the woman's immune system that allow her to carry the baby inside her body (NINDS, 2009). Other studies have found few relationships between MS symptoms and pregnancy and no links between pregnancy and the course of disease. Importantly, women with MS do not experience worse birth outcomes (such as miscarriages, ectopic pregnancies, or stillbirths) than other women.

The major threat to the child developing in utero is the possibility of birth defects caused by certain drugs used to treat MS (see Chapter 6). Although no human data are available, animal studies suggest that drugs that are treatment mainstays of MS, including corticosteroids and interferon beta, can harm the fetus during gestation. Therefore, women with MS who are thinking about becoming pregnant may need to either stop or change their MS treatments if the drug they are taking carries risks of fetal anomalies.

DIAGNOSING MS

The symptoms associated with MS are multiple and varied, and each traces back directly to one or more lesions in the central nervous system. The clinical history—the patient's experiences with symptoms over time—and neurological examination remain the most important factors in diagnosing MS, despite the development of MRI (magnetic resonance imaging) technology (see Chapter 2) and its impressive images. The diagnosis of MS requires that patients have lesions affecting multiple (two or more) areas of the central nervous system and that these lesions occur more than once (two or more times). Although no individual symptoms are unique to MS (all the symptoms that persons with MS experience also occur in other diseases), certain types of problems are highly characteristic of the disease (see Table 5.1). Thus, the typical MS patient is a young adult (between 15 and 50 years old) who has one or more of the following characteristic symptoms at two or more points in time, typically with complete resolution of the symptoms between these episodes:

- Optic neuritis or other visual symptoms,
- Lhermitte's sign,
- Fatigue,

- Heat sensitivity, or
- Sensory abnormalities.

Because these symptoms are nonspecific (not unique to MS), neurologists typically perform other tests before making a final diagnosis of MS (Olek, 2008b). As described in Chapter 2, the availability of MRI scanning beginning in the 1980s fundamentally transformed the diagnosis of MS. As shown in Figure 5.3, a schematic drawing suggesting typical findings of a brain MRI scan of a patient with disseminated MS plaques, the plaques caused by myelin destruction (see Chapter 4) light up as white so-called bright spots against the dense grey appearance of normal brain tissues.

Researchers have found ways to enhance the ability of MRI to detect MS plaques, especially those with inflammation around the lesions. This enhancement requires injecting patients with a contrast agent involving gadolinium (a magnetic, metallic element of the rare-earth group, with the symbol *Gd* in the table of elements) shortly before they have their MRI scans. Gadolinium-enhanced MRI scans are especially useful for discovering fresh MS plaques and for monitoring MS activity in the brain and the spinal cord. New MRI techniques, such as magnetization transfer imaging and diffusion-tensor MRI, might improve the ability of MRI to detect subtle lesions in the future (NINDS, 2009).

Despite its immense benefits, MRI is not perfectly accurate at diagnosing MS: approximately 80 to 90 percent of persons with MS have abnormal MRI scans (Olek, 2008b). Furthermore, other diseases can produce similar MRI findings to

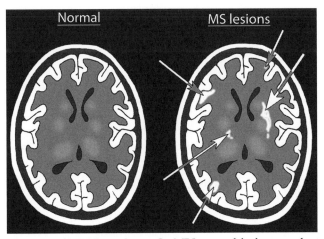

Figure 5.3. Drawing of MRI Brain Scans. On MRI scans of the brains and spinal cords of persons with MS, areas of MS plaques show up as bright white spots. [Anil Shukla]

those seen in MS. Therefore, in addition to MRI, neurologists use other tests to provide more evidence to confirm the diagnosis. Since the mid-twentieth century, neurologists have performed lumbar punctures to obtain CSF for analysis, as described in Chapter 2. Electrophoresis analysis of CSF can identify specific patterns of immunoglobulin G antibodies suggestive of MS. As shown in Figure 5.4, the so-called oligoclonal pattern occurs when specific immune globulins migrate together on the electrophoresis medium to produce several closely spaced bands (olig means few; clonal in this context means a group of replicas or clones of a large molecule). From 85 to 95 percent of persons with MS show oligoclonal banding of their CSF.

Other common tests involve what are called evoked potentials—a measure of the time required to produce an electrical response in the brain after stimulating specific parts of the body. In evoked potential testing, technicians tape electrodes, cushioned with a dollop of conducting gel, to the patient's scalp; the

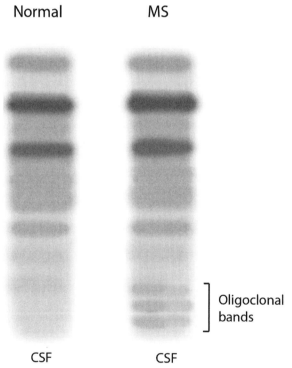

Figure 5.4. Oligoclonal Bands in the CSF. Electrophoresis analysis of CSF identifies specific patterns of immunoglobulin G antibodies suggestive of MS. The oligoclonal pattern occurs when specific immune globulins migrate together to produce several closely spaced bands. [Anil Shukla]

positioning of these electrodes on the head depends on the part of the body being tested. For example, when the test is studying the brain's response to visual stimulation, the technician applies the electrodes to the back of the head over the occipital region of the brain, which processes visual images. Sensitive instruments record the brain waves detected by the electrodes after the nerve stimulation. The time between the stimulation and the brain's electrical response is called the latency, and it indicates the speed with which nerves conduct their signals (see Chapter 1). If the nerve conduction speed is slower than normal, the test suggests the diagnosis of MS. Three types of evoked potential testing are commonly performed in diagnostic work-ups of MS (Olek, 2008b):

- Visual evoked potentials, in which patients' eyes (and thus the nerves involved in conducting visual images) are stimulated by a strobe light or checkerboard pattern on a screen: 85 percent of persons with definite MS have abnormal results.
- Brain stem auditory evoked potentials, in which patients' ears (nerves involved in processing sounds) are stimulated by clicking noises or test tones through earphones: 67 percent of persons with definite MS have abnormal results.
- Somatosensory evoked potentials, in which patients' arms or legs (sensory and motor nerves) are stimulated by mild electrical shocks administered to the wrist or knee: 77 percent of persons with definite MS have abnormal results.

Even patients without obvious symptoms involving the nerves tested can have abnormal evoked potential tests. For example, someone who describes no difficulty hearing can nonetheless have abnormal brain stem auditory evoked potentials. Furthermore, as with other diagnostic testing in MS, other neurological conditions can cause abnormal evoked potentials.

Given the complexities of these diagnostic evaluations, only time will tell if someone with new symptoms and various test results truly has MS. All the sophisticated and expensive diagnostic testing may not produce a definitive diagnosis. Nevertheless, even though patients might have trouble putting their eerie and sometimes ephemeral symptoms into words, listening carefully as patients describe their bodily experiences may provide virtually all the evidence a skilled neurologist needs to diagnose MS. The symptoms over time largely tell the story.

6

MS Treatments

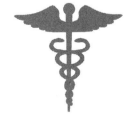

MS has no cure. For more than 250 years, doctors and patients have tried numerous and varied therapies to relieve symptoms and stem the disabling effects of MS, but with little or time-limited success. Today's treatments have certainly advanced beyond the myriad and generally fruitless interventions of the nineteenth and early twentieth centuries described in Chapter 2. But without precisely understanding what causes the disease—and what produces the differing patterns of illness—designing treatments that target the roots of MS is challenging.

Nonetheless, increasing knowledge about the pathology of MS lesions (see Chapter 1) and the role of the immune system in the disease (see Chapter 4) has led to significant therapeutic advancements in the last 20 years. Nowadays, neurologists can offer persons newly diagnosed with MS medications that can slow progression of the disease—but only for some patients and for limited periods of time. Since the early 1990s, these treatments have provided important benefits (such as reduced disability and fewer relapses) to certain persons with MS, which last for several years or sometimes longer.

These important new treatments, however, carry significant costs in terms of side effects. Individual patients therefore must weigh the risks (side effects) versus the benefits (possibly slowing disease progression) of these therapies and make treatment decisions based on their own personal preferences. Their decision making is complicated by the inability to predict, up front, which patients will benefit from these treatments. In other words, there is no perfect clairvoyance—no proverbial crystal ball—to guide treatment decisions for individual patients.

Persons with MS today receive different treatments depending on their therapeutic goals:

1. Treating an acute MS flare to restore patients to their baseline functioning (to get patients back to a comparable physical state as before their MS flare or exacerbation);
2. Slowing disease progression or modifying the course of MS to make it less disabling; or
3. Treating a sign or symptom of MS, such as optic neuritis (eye problems), muscle spasticity, bladder or bowel problems, fatigue, pain, or cognitive difficulties (see Chapter 5).

The approaches for addressing each of these three therapeutic goals vary. The treatments can involve medications taken either orally as pills (ingested and absorbed through the digestive tract) or parenterally (introduced into the bloodstream by methods other than through the digestive tract), typically by intravenous infusion (fluid injected through a thin tubing inserted into a vein), intramuscular injection (injection into a muscle), or subcutaneous injection (injection just under the skin but above the muscle). Other interventions include rehabilitation therapies (see Chapter 7) or assistive technologies, such as ambulation aids (canes, crutches, or walkers) and wheelchairs (see Chapter 8).

This chapter focuses on the drugs or medications used to address the three broad therapeutic goals (treating flares, slowing disease progression, and treating signs and symptoms). The chapter concludes by examining briefly so-called complementary and alternative therapies: treatments considered outside mainstream, traditional Western medicine but used by many persons with MS. Before beginning, it is important to note that research on MS treatments is very active. By the time this book is published, a brand new medication may have transformed the therapeutic landscape and have begun offering hope to hundreds of thousands of persons with MS.

However, the phrase caveat emptor—buyer beware—is highly relevant to MS therapeutics, where new drug discoveries or supposed advances are announced multiple times each year. Excited stories appear in newspapers, on the television, or on Internet blogs and Web sites, touting the latest advance in MS treatments and making grandiose claims of success. With few exceptions, reports rarely appear later after the much hyped therapeutic breakthrough fails to show sustained benefits over time. A major challenge to demonstrating the benefits of MS treatments is the need to track patients from year to year to assess how they are doing. Drugs that show some short-term advantage may turn out to offer little improvement over time.

In the mid-1980s, shortly after I was diagnosed with MS, a young but nevertheless wise neurologist gave me a warning. He predicted that, in the years ahead, people would frequently approach me brandishing the latest newspaper article claiming a dramatic breakthrough in MS treatment. Excited and hopeful, they would exhort me to give it a try. Be cautious, he urged. Wait a little while; see what later research studies show about the therapeutic benefits versus side effects; make your own choices based on what works best for you, how you want to approach your lifelong disease. Don't be swayed by hype that might lead to later disappointment. He was absolutely right!

TREATING MS FLARES

During flares of MS (also called relapses, attacks, or acute exacerbations), persons experience relatively sudden and disabling functional impairments. When flares occur, treatment aims to shorten the exacerbation and return the person to baseline functioning (functional levels comparable to their status before the flare) as soon as possible (Olek, 2008d; NINDS, 2009). Neurologists typically do not treat flares unless there is clinical evidence of new disease activity, such as loss of vision, motor problems (muscle weakness), or symptoms suggesting lesions in the cerebellum region of the brain (imbalance). Some neurologists also require that a new lesion, associated anatomically with the new sign or symptom, be visible on an MRI scan.

Neurologists may not recommend treating flares involving purely sensory symptoms, such as sharp pains or searing burning sensations. Instead, they would try analgesia to treat the pain itself. Evidence suggests that the usual treatment for MS flares is less effective for sensory compared with other symptoms, such as motor problems. In addition, treatments can have significant side effects.

Glucocorticoids

Glucocorticoids are the mainstay of treatment for MS flares. Encompassing a range of specific chemical compounds, glucocorticoids are a type of steroid (specifically, corticosteroids) that plays roles in metabolism of carbohydrates, proteins, and fats and also have other important biological functions. In particular, glucocorticoids have anti-inflammatory and immunosuppressive effects: they combat inflammation and its consequences and suppress immune system activities. The benefits of glucocorticoids in resolving acute MS exacerbations likely result from these combined anti-inflammatory and immunosuppressive effects. Corticosteroids may also bolster the blood-brain barrier, making it more difficult for immune system cells circulating in the peripheral blood to enter the central nervous system and attack brain tissues (see Figure 4.1).

Cortisol, the natural glucocorticoid, is produced by the outer cortex (region) of the adrenal glands, which sit atop the kidneys. Adrenocorticotropic hormone (ACTH), released by the anterior pituitary gland in the brain, regulates cortisol production. Secretion of ACTH is itself regulated by the corticotropin-releasing hormone, a polypeptide (molecular chain of amino acids) discharged by the hypothalamus part of the brain in response to signals released by the nervous system. Cortisol rises in the peripheral blood when persons experience physical or psychological stresses. Along with releases of adrenaline, another adrenal gland hormone, cortisol surges support the fight-or-flight reaction: the body's natural response to confronting danger or stress. Elevated cortisol increases glucose (sugar) levels in the bloodstream, heightens the brain's glucose consumption, and down regulates (turns off) biological functions (such as the digestive system) that would compete with the body's focus on fighting a foe.

To treat MS flares, patients receive either synthetic glucocorticoids or ACTH, which stimulates natural cortisol production. Synthetic glucocorticoids come in various forms, specifically the drugs prednisone, prednisolone, methylprednisolone, betamethasone, and dexamethasone. Some, like prednisone, are taken as pills, while others require parenteral administration. ACTH is administered by injection.

Studies suggest that glucocorticoids significantly shorten the length of MS flares and return persons to baseline functional status, but there is no evidence that these compounds reduce long-term disability or improve the course of disease. Neurologists debate the details of how best to use glucocorticoids in treating MS flares. Intravenous methylprednisolone seems to be more effective than ACTH or oral prednisone, but the circumstances of individual patients may dictate the appropriate drug regimen. Intravenous administration generally involves infusions of high doses of methylprednisolone daily, across four or five days. Infusions typically take place in outpatient clinics, although it is sometimes possible to arrange intravenous treatments in the home (such as with a visiting nurse).

Patients may not sense improvements in their impairments until a month or six weeks after medication ends. Therefore, patients must have patience after their infusions or pill treatments conclude, awaiting gradual restoration of their baseline functioning. Given the naturally waxing and waning nature of relapsing-remitting MS, this raises the question of whether glucocorticoid treatment really did the trick: or did the patient's condition improve on its own? Studies comparing glucocorticoid to placebo (sugar pills or salt water infusions) have shown significant benefits from glucocorticoids in resolving acute exacerbations. Therefore, experts believe that glucocorticoid treatment is beneficial in shortening flares, with about 90 percent of patients showing improvement.

Glucocorticoids are powerful compounds, and they have significant side effects. Taking high doses of synthetic glucocorticoids or ACTH can suppress natural adrenal gland production of cortisol, which as noted above is a critical stress hormone. Some physicians prescribe low, short-term doses of prednisone as a so-called taper following intravenous glucocorticoid administration, to ease the transition back to the natural balance. Other physicians do not believe a prednisone taper is required after short courses of high-dose steroids. Long-term or repeated use of steroids can contribute to thinning of the bones or osteoporosis.

Other immediate side effects of glucocorticoids include sleep disturbances, weight gain, puffiness, and changes in mood. In particular, steroids can precipitate agitation and emotional mood swings, from euphoria to depression. Sometimes, steroid-induced mood alterations can become very frightening. Physicians must warn patients about these side effects beforehand so they are not surprised by their occurrence and know when to consult their doctors if side effects become troubling.

Plasma Exchange

Glucocorticoids do not resolve acute exacerbations in approximately 10 percent of patients. Plasma exchange is an intensive treatment, which aims to remove antibodies circulating in the blood from the body under the assumption that these antibodies have contributed to the immune process that precipitated the flare (see Figure 4.1). Plasma is the liquid portion of the blood. Red blood cells (erythrocytes), white blood cells (granulocytes and lymphocytes, among others), and platelets travel throughout arteries and veins floating in plasma. Other compounds, such as the potentially offending antibodies, are also dispersed in plasma.

Plasma exchange, also known as plasmapheresis, involves three steps:

1. A thin tube is inserted into a vein, and whole blood is withdrawn from a patient and directed to flow into the plasma exchange machine;
2. Through a very fine filtration process, the machine separates the liquid or plasma from the red and white blood cells and platelets and replaces it with fresh, clean liquid; and

3. The reconstituted blood, with its red and white blood cells and platelets floating in the replacement plasma, is transfused back into the patient.

Plasma exchange is an effective treatment in diseases where antibodies circulating in peripheral blood are clearly destructive, such as myasthenia gravis and Guillain-Barré syndrome, two autoimmune conditions. Neurologists have speculated that, since autoimmune processes might cause MS lesions (see Chapter 4), plasmapheresis might also benefit MS patients. Thus far, studies have provided contradictory evidence about whether plasma exchange improves long-term functioning in patients with progressive MS. However, plasma exchange might shorten acute exacerbations.

Since about 90 percent of patients with MS flares respond to glucocorticoids, experts do not recommend plasma exchange for individuals with acute exacerbations. Instead, physicians should reserve plasmapheresis for severely impaired patients who fail to improve from glucocorticoid treatments. Potential side effects from plasma exchange include blood clotting problems and infections.

DISEASE-MODIFYING MEDICATIONS

In 1993, the U.S. Food and Drug Administration approved the first medication that might slow the course of MS. This event fundamentally transformed the approach toward treating newly diagnosed individuals with the relapsing-remitting pattern of disease. The first of these so-called disease-modifying medications or agents was interferon beta-1b, which is sold under the brand name Betaseron®. By 2006, six drugs had gained approval (see Table 6.1). To obtain Food and Drug Administration approval, drugs must undergo rigorous clinical trial testing and prove that they are safe and effective for the desired use. Unlike the glucocorticoids discussed above, which aim to treat MS only when the disease flares up, the exciting goal of these new medications was to stop, slow, or delay exacerbations and the progressive disability caused by MS.

All six disease-modifying drugs affect the immune system in some, albeit slightly different, ways. Given their focus on modulating the immune responses, starting these drugs early, shortly after diagnoses, becomes critical (Olek, 2008f; National Multiple Sclerosis Society, 2009). As described in Chapter 4, immunological processes probably play their primary destructive role in the first few years of active MS. After that, degeneration takes greater precedence, with progressive deterioration of the cellular integrity of neurons and axons and replacement by fibrosis. These degraded cells no longer function normally. Some experts believe

Table 6.1
Disease-Modifying Medications

Generic Name	Brand Name	Approval Date[a]	Mode of Administration
Interferon beta-1b	Betaseron®	1993	Subcutaneous injection every other day
Interferon beta-1a	Avonex®	1996	Intramuscular injection once a week
Glatiramer acetate	Copaxone®	1996	Subcutaneous injection every day
Mitoxantrone	Novantrone®[b]	2000	Intravenous infusion 4 times a year; lifetime limit of 8–12 doses
Interferon beta-1a	Rebif®	2002	Subcutaneous injection 3 times a week
Natalizumab	Tysabri®	2006	Intravenous infusion every 4 weeks in registered facility

[a]Year the U.S. Food and Drug Administration approved the drug for use in MS.
[b]As of 2006, a generic version of mitoxantrone became available.

that degeneration of neurons actually begins very early, even as the autoimmune destruction is at its height.

Given this mechanism of action (mode of working) of today's disease-modifying medications, practice guidelines advise neurologists to offer all patients newly diagnosed with MS one of these drugs. As described below, experts advise starting with one of the interferons or glatiramer acetate and holding natalizumab and mitoxantrone in reserve, in case patients continue to experience acute exacerbations. The latter two drugs have more complicated and serious side effect profiles.

Each of the disease-modifying medications can have significant side effects and requires parenteral administration, multiple times a week for three of the drugs. Individual patients need to choose for themselves their willingness to tolerate possible side effects and the lifestyle implications of using these powerful injectable drugs. Patients' decisions are complicated by the fact that—as noted at the beginning of this chapter—these drugs do not work for everyone and the benefits may not persist over time. Substantial fractions of patients will continue to experience progressive disability while on these disease-modifying medications, although this progression may be slower than without the drug. Unfortunately, there is no way to predict whether a given drug will benefit a specific patient.

Interferon Beta

Interferons are compounds produced naturally by the human body to combat infections, such as viruses. Interferons come in three major types:

- Interferon alpha, produced by different white blood cells and capable of stopping viruses from replicating, cells from proliferating, and regulating immune responses; it is used to treat certain types of cancers and leukemia;
- Interferon gamma, produced by the T cells that regulate the immune response; it is used to treat rheumatoid arthritis, some cancers, and other immunological diseases; and it might contribute to MS autoimmune activity; and
- Interferon beta, produced by fibroblasts (cells that generate the matrix structure surrounding connective tissues); it has antiviral activity, as well as the ability to affect immune system responses.

Interferon beta is produced for commercial purposes using sophisticated biotechnological manufacturing techniques, which differ for interferon beta-1a versus beta-1b.

No one knows exactly how interferon beta works to slow MS progression, although the compound's anti-inflammatory actions may play a role. Another possibility is that interferon beta blocks the action of immune cells, such as activated T lymphocytes, perhaps blocking passage through the blood-brain barrier (see Figure 6.1). Yet another conjecture is that interferon beta acts by inhibiting interferon gamma, which might contribute to MS attacks.

Different interferon products have varying administration regimens, requiring injections from one to three times per week (see Table 6.1). The three drugs seem to have similar levels of benefit in slowing disease progression and reducing rates of attacks, although the strongest evidence suggests that these benefits may last perhaps only for a year or two. Earlier studies tracking patients' outcomes over time had serious methodological limitations. More recent research presents stronger evidence about the long-term benefits and risks of treatment.

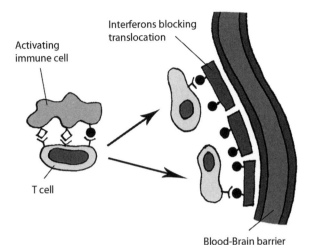

Figure 6.1. One Possible Way Interferon Beta Works. Experts do not know exactly how interferon beta works in MS. One possibility is that the drug blocks passage of activated immune cells across the blood-brain barrier and into the central nervous system. [Anil Shukla]

The interferons beta can have significant side effects, although side effect profiles differ slightly across the medication types and vary widely across individual patients. Interferons should not be taken during pregnancy because of potential risks to the developing fetus. Common interferon beta side effects include the following:

- Irritation at the injection site, such as swelling, redness, and pain; severe skin damage including necrosis (tissue death) occurs in a small fraction of patients
- Flu-like symptoms for a day or two after drug administration, marked by chills, fever, muscle aches, sweating, and fatigue
- Allergic reactions that can be severe, interfering with breathing
- Heightened risk of seizures, including more frequent seizures among individuals with known seizure disorders and new seizures for those without a seizure history
- Liver abnormalities, which are generally mild but can be more serious; interferon beta-1a now carries a warning about the possibility of severe liver damage
- Lower blood counts, including lower levels of red and white blood cells and platelets
- Mood disturbances, including depression, sadness, anxiety, difficulty sleeping, and irritability

Another problem is the development of neutralizing antibodies—the body's production of antibodies (see Chapter 4) to interferon beta. Neutralizing antibodies limit the effectiveness of interferon beta in treating MS. The likelihood of developing neutralizing antibodies differs across the three interferon beta medications, and it also varies based on the dosages of drugs, periodicity of use (once a week versus three times weekly), and length of use. Some patients revert spontaneously to become free of these neutralizing antibodies, allowing the interferon beta to become active once again. The complexities surrounding neutralizing antibody development complicate decisions about which interferon beta regimen to use.

Glatiramer Acetate

Glatiramer acetate is a synthetic protein (specifically random polymers of four amino acids) that mimics myelin basic protein, a major component of the myelin sheath that protects neuronal axons and is a target of autoimmune attack in MS (see Chapter 4). Through some mechanism that remains unclear, glatiramer acetate blocks the destructive action of activated T lymphocytes. It may act as a decoy or supplant myelin basic protein as a target for T cell attacks. In addition, glatiramer acetate seems to induce other T cells that serve to suppress the immune response in the central nervous system.

Glatiramer acetate requires daily subcutaneous injection. In a placebo-controlled study, glatiramer acetate produced significantly lower relapse rates and disease progression than did the placebo. The side effect profile of glatiramer acetate is less extensive than for the interferons beta. Persons can experience irritation and soreness at the injection site. A small fraction of patients develop acute post-injection sensations, including chest tightness, heart palpitations, anxiety, and breathing difficulties. Although these sensations are scary, they typically resolve within 15 minutes and do not happen again. Although negative effects on a developing fetus may be less than for the interferons beta, women who become pregnant typically should not start or continue glatiramer acetate. Although neutralizing antibodies may develop to glatiramer, they do not impede drug action as they do for the interferons beta.

Mitoxantrone

Mitoxantrone was developed originally to treat cancers; in 2000, it was approved for use in MS. Mitoxantrone acts by inhibiting the activity of T cells, B cells, and macrophages in autoimmune attacks on myelin sheaths. It is a powerful immunosuppressive medication. Mitoxantrone has substantial side effects, including a small risk of developing leukemia (specifically acute myelogenous leukemia). The most notable risk is cardiac (heart) toxicity. Because of dangers of damaging the heart, persons with MS are limited in the total amount of mitoxantrone they can receive over their lifetimes. Typically, persons can receive up to 4 intravenous infusions of mitoxantrone per year, for a total of 8 to 12 dosages across two to three years. Persons with documented heart disease should not receive mitoxantrone.

Although mitoxantrone may produce small benefits in slowing MS disability, its toxicities may overtake these modest benefits. Therefore, neurologists typically reserve mitoxantrone for patients whose MS is progressing rapidly and who have failed to benefit from other disease-modifying medications. After mitoxantrone treatment, persons should try to avoid contact with persons with infectious diseases. With immune systems suppressed by the mitoxantrone, succumbing to an overwhelming infection becomes a significant risk.

Natalizumab

Natalizumab is the most recent disease-modifying medication to win approval from the U.S. Food and Drug Administration, but its introduction had a rocky start. The Internet was abuzz with anticipation before the introduction of natalizumab in the fall of 2004. This drug, produced by recombinant techniques (genetic engineering), represented a novel immunological approach. Natalizumab is a monoclonal antibody directed against alpha-4 integrins: proteins expressed on the surfaces of inflammatory lymphocytes that promote their binding to the surface of blood vessels (specifically binding to the vascular endothelium). Natalizumab appears to impede passage of inflammatory lymphocytes across the blood-brain barrier, where they can damage tissues in the central nervous system.

Early studies randomly assigned MS patients with relapsing-remitting MS to receive either natalizumab or a placebo. These studies found that patients treated with natalizumab had significantly less disability at two years of follow-up compared with those receiving the placebo. In addition, patients receiving natalizumab appeared to report significantly better health–related quality of life. The results were no better than those found in comparable studies involving interferon beta or glatiramer acetate. The novelty of the monoclonal antibody and specificity of its immunological target, however, generated excitement among MS patients and their advocates.

Several months after its introduction, reports emerged of two deaths of patients receiving natalizumab; in February 2005, the manufacturer withdrew the drug from the market. The patients had died from a rare neurological disease called progressive multifocal leukoencephalopathy or PML. The PML was caused by reactivation of an infection by a virus known as the JC virus, based on the initials (J. C.) of the patient from whom the virus had first been isolated about 35 years previously. JC viral loads rise in the serum (the watery portion of blood plasma) after initiation of natalizumab treatment and before onset of the PML symptoms, suggesting a link between natalizumab and the PML deaths.

For the next year, natalizumab's manufacturer continued studying health outcomes of patients taking the drug, finding no more deaths. The company estimated PML deaths from the drug at roughly 1 per 1,000 patients who had taken natalizumab for an average of 18 months. In February 2006, the Food and Drug Administration lifted its suspension on natalizumab, and in June 2006, it approved the drug's use as a solo therapy (not to be used in combination with other disease-modifying medications) for relapsing forms of MS. In June 2008, two more PML deaths of MS patients taking natalizumab were announced, but the drug remained on the market.

Natalizumab may be associated with other serious side effects besides the rare but lethal PML. Early reports suggested possible increased risk of melanoma, a dangerous form of skin cancer. In February 2008, the manufacturer reported instances of significant liver damage. All these concerns have prompted neurologists to proceed cautiously in recommending natalizumab to their patients. Guidelines released by the American Academy of Neurology recommend that natalizumab be given only to patients whose MS is progressing despite other disease-modifying medications or who are unable to tolerate the other drugs. Furthermore, patients may receive the monthly natalizumab intravenous infusions only at centers around the United States that are specifically trained and approved to provide the drug.

Medication Costs

"If you take these drugs for multiple sclerosis," said MS expert T. Jock Murray (Moore, 2002), "we can show that your attacks are less frequent, that the severity is less, and your MRI will improve. The implication is that in the future, you'll be better off. That's not clear." Dr. Murray stirred up particular controversy when he looked at the costs of disease-modifying medications, which then in his native Canada averaged $17,000 per year. He and his colleagues estimated that it would cost $170,000 over 10 years to reduce MS exacerbations by only one-third, the supposed effectiveness of the medications known at that time. In particular, it would cost about $47,000 to eliminate a single MS flare.

In the United States, the costs of MS disease-modifying medications range from $15,000 to nearly $30,000 per year. Part of this expense relates to the high cost of drug development and advertising and the fact that most disease-modifying drugs are not yet generic. Generic versions of drugs are chemically identical to those of the brand name drug, but they are manufactured by other companies that have not borne the original costs of drug development and thus can sell the drug more cheaply. (To allow pharmaceutical companies to recoup their investments in developing new drugs, the U.S. government grants them patent protections for up to 20 years after the drug's invention.) While health insurance often pays at least a portion of these drug costs—and there are specific nongovernmental programs that support medication expenses for some persons with MS—these drugs represent a huge expense with often unproven long-term benefits for individual patients. Other less appreciated costs involve the expense of treating potential drug side effects.

How much money is it worth spending to give someone with MS a disease-modifying medication? This remains an open societal question. The answer to this question will depend on one's perspective. Patients and family members will likely have different points of view than do executives of health insurance companies, which bear the costs, or health policy makers thinking about distribution of scarce health dollars across populations. Similarly, patients who have done well and experienced few side effects from the medications will have different perceptions from those of patients who have suffered serious ill effects. Perhaps the largest impediment to answering this question objectively remains the query at the core of Dr. Murray's commentary. We still do not know how disease-modifying medications affect the functional impairments and disability caused by MS over the long term.

TREATING OTHER FORMS OF MS

The disease-modifying medications discussed above are prescribed generally only for persons with relapsing-remitting patterns of disease. Studies of interferon beta and glatiramer acetate in secondary progressive MS—the pattern eventually experienced by about 80 percent of persons who begin with relapsing-remitting MS—have shown little benefit. Nonetheless, these drugs might offer some benefit to patients who experience acute exacerbations on top of their secondary progressive declines. To try to prevent or limit these attacks, some neurologists recommend interferon beta for their patients with secondary progressive MS. Mitoxantrone might reduce progression for persons with severely deteriorating functioning, but the cardiac toxicity of this drug significantly limits its utility, as described above. None of the disease-modifying medications appear to benefit persons with primary progressive MS.

Neurologists have experimented with numerous other medications for both secondary and primary progressive MS (Olek, 2008e). Overall, the results parallel the general experience of MS therapeutics: no drugs prevent declines although some medications may assist certain patients for limited periods of time. The most common medication recommendations for persons with secondary progressive MS include the following:

- Monthly intravenous infusions of a single, high dose of methylprednisolone, the same glucocorticoid frequently used to treat MS flares (see above). This monthly intravenous dose is also known as a monthly pulse or bolus of methylprednisolone. Research evidence supporting this approach is scanty, but some neurologists believe it can delay progression of impairments.
- Monthly glucocorticoid pulses combined with intravenous cyclophosphamide, an anticancer medication that also has immunosuppressive actions. Cyclophosphamide is a synthetic alkylating agent (a compound that introduces alkyl molecules to other compounds), which is chemically related to the nitrogen mustards (various toxic compounds). This approach may benefit younger patients more than older individuals, but again strong evidence of beneficial effects is lacking.
- Methotrexate, either taken orally or through a subcutaneous injection. Methotrexate, which affects immune system function, is also used to treat certain cancers, rheumatoid arthritis, and other autoimmune conditions. Strong evidence of benefit is also sparse.

The options for treatment of primary progressive MS are even more limited. Neurologists recommend regimens similar to those for secondary progressive MS, such as monthly methylprednisolone pulses and methotrexate. In cases of severe functional declines, mitoxantrone may be worth trying, recognizing its cardiac toxicity. Cladribine, a potent immunosuppressive medication that is used in treating certain leukemias, may have some albeit limited benefit. Little, thus far, has slowed the functional impairments of primary progressive MS.

NEW AREAS OF RESEARCH IN MS TREATMENT

Considerable research is under way exploring new ways to treat MS (NINDS, 2009). Several promising areas of research are addressing different points of the pathological process that causes MS (see Chapters 1 and 4). Even once a new approach is found, however, it can take many years to determine whether the treatment is safe and effective for use in persons with MS. Furthermore, as noted throughout this chapter, since MS is currently a lifelong disease, truly beneficial treatments must produce long-term or sustained functional improvements. Examples of active areas of investigation are described below.

Stimulating Remyelination

As described in Chapters 1 and 4, MS lesions occur when the myelin sheaths produced by oligodendrocytes deteriorate and no longer insulate neuronal axons. Scientists have learned that oligodendrocytes can indeed multiply and lay down new myelin after an attack. Research is exploring whether various medications may either stimulate or inhibit this remyelination.

Improving Nerve Conduction

Damage of the myelin sheath impairs conduction of electrical impulses down nerve axons in the central nervous system, leading to the varied disabling consequences of MS. Degeneration of the nerves also slows impulse conduction. Researchers are therefore trying to find ways to speed the passage of electrical impulses in nerves damaged by MS.

One target involves potassium ions, which behave abnormally along nerve axons impaired by MS. Drugs that block the channels through which potassium ions flow into and out of nerve cells show promise of improving impulse conduction. Several small studies have shown that drugs playing this role (derivatives of aminopyridine) improve vision, strength, and coordination but with some side effects. Ongoing research is examining various strategies for enhancing nerve conduction.

Cytokines

Researchers are investigating the roles of various different cytokines (proteins that are produced by T cells and regulate the immune system) in the development and progression of MS. Interferons are cytokines, but there are many other types. In mice with a condition similar to MS, a cytokine called interleukin-4 can reduce demyelination and improve physical functioning. Interleukin-4 appears to work by making T cells protect rather than destroy myelin. Scientists are considering ways to enhance the beneficial effects of interleukin-4 and other similar compounds.

Vaccines

Researchers are exploring creation of a vaccine to prevent myelin destruction. Vaccine development involves extracting T cells that attack myelin from patients' blood, inactivating them, and injecting them back into mice with a condition that mimics MS (experimental allergic encephalomyelitis or EAE). This procedure resulted in destruction of the immune system's cells that were attacking the mice's myelin. Researchers have tested a similar vaccine approach in humans, but the numbers of persons tested were small and it is much too soon to know whether this method will prevent or slow myelin destruction. One impediment to developing vaccines is that T cells vary significantly from person to person. Developing a single vaccine—or even a series of vaccines—that would benefit most patients presents enormous challenges.

Peptide Therapy

The notion underlying peptide therapy is based on observing that the body can produce an immune response against the T cells that are destroying myelin, but that this immune response is fairly weak and thus does not stop the destruction. To bolster the immune response against the rogue T cells, researchers study the myelin-destroying T cells to identify the receptor on their surface that recognizes myelin. They then use biotechnology techniques to create this receptor outside the animal's body and afterward inject a fragment of this receptor back into the animal. The animal's immune system recognizes this fragment as a foreign invader and launches an intensive attack against any cells carrying this fragment: the myelin-destroying T cells. Peptide therapy thus stimulates the body's immune system to stop its own destructive cells.

Stem Cell Transplants

Stem cells are precursor or undifferentiated cells that give rise to all cells throughout the body. In particular, hematopoietic stem cells produce all the cells involved in the immune system and the cells that circulate in the blood. Hematopoietic stem cells live mostly in the bone marrow, but some also find their way into the blood stream. In autologous stem cell transplants, a person's own stem cells are taken out of his or her circulating blood, separated from other cells (such as red and white blood cells), and returned to the person's bloodstream through an intravenous infusion. The goal of autologous stem cell transplantation is to suppress the immune system, which has become self-destructive in MS.

Stem cell transplantation carries many risks, including death. Studies have thus far shown mixed results, without conclusive evidence of benefit. More clinical trials of stem cell transplantation in MS are ongoing.

MEDICATIONS FOR MS SIGNS AND SYMPTOMS

Another major goal of therapy is to treat the signs and symptoms of MS, which can have such negative consequences on daily functional abilities and quality of life. As described in Chapter 5, MS can affect a wide range of bodily processes and activities, quite literally from head to toe. Rehabilitation therapy can assist persons with a variety of issues, such as physical therapy to address weakness, spasticity, impaired balance, and other physical deficits; occupational therapy to help with cognitive dysfunction and problems performing activities of daily living; and speech-language therapy to address speech problems and swallowing difficulties (see Chapter 7). Mobility aids become necessary when persons cannot walk safely and independently (see Chapter 8). The discussion below highlights medication treatments for several major problems caused by MS. Drugs and other treatments are also available for additional problems related to MS, including pain, depression, sexual dysfunction, and seizures.

Spasticity

Spasticity can cause significant problems for persons with MS, causing the legs to extend involuntarily and sometimes even raising a person's upper body from his or her bed. Spasticity is generally worse in the legs than the arms. While physical therapy can be useful especially for preventing muscle shortening and contractures (permanent shortening of muscles, producing deformities), medications offer critical benefits. Drugs for treating spasticity include baclofen, tizanidine, and dantrolene, although each can have side effects, such as dry mouth, drowsiness, and motor weakness.

If spasticity is severe and does not respond to oral medications, baclofen can be infused directly into the central nervous system through an intrathecal pump. This small device pumps the baclofen directly into the space underneath the arachnoid membrane in the spinal cord (see Chapter 1). Because implantable pumps can cause complications, this approach should be used only in persons whose spasticity fails to respond to oral medications.

Fatigue

The majority of persons with MS experience profound fatigue at some time. This overwhelming exhaustion can be present upon awakening and worsen during the day but without obvious relationship to the activities performed. Heat can worsen fatigue. Common sense remedies include remaining in air-conditioned spaces during hot summer days and avoiding becoming overheated. Depression can contribute to fatigue and needs attention and treatment. Physicians should also evaluate patients for treatable causes of fatigue, such as anemia, thyroid problems, and certain medications (such as antihistamines and selected heart medicines).

If persons remain exhausted from their MS, medications might help. One option is amantadine, which was originally developed to treat influenza A. During early drug testing, amantadine was also found to benefit persons with Parkinson's disease, another degenerative neurological condition. Amantadine passes easily across the blood-brain barrier into the central nervous system. Although how it works remains unclear, amantadine reduces fatigue in persons with MS. The drug's side effects include a very dry mouth. If persons do not respond to amantadine, pemoline is another medication option.

Bladder and Bowel Problems

MS can significantly affect bladder and bowel function, typically to the same degree as a person's motor weakness. The major bowel problem is constipation, and no prescription drug can solve this difficulty. Eating a high fiber diet and drinking fluids are common sense responses. Persons can also use over-the-counter preparations (stool softeners and mild laxatives) to maintain bowel regularity. Unfortunately, drinking fluids to facilitate bowel functioning may cause problems with bladder control.

Bladder dysfunction requires thorough evaluation, since the appropriate treatment depends on the nature of the problem. Patients learn early on to control their fluid intake and take frequent restroom breaks to avoid episodes of urinary incontinence. For some patients, cranberry juice can alter urine chemistry and help prevent urinary tract infections, which exacerbate urinary urgency. If patients are unable to void their bladder and retain large amounts of urine, they may require mechanical assistance: inserting a narrow catheter (plastic tube) through the urethra into the bladder to allow the fluid to drain out by gravity. These patients must perform urinary catheterization several times a day and maintain excellent hygiene to prevent development of dangerous urinary tract infections. For men, frequent urinary catheterization can damage the prostate gland. Different medications are available to help patients in whom urinary urgency and incontinence are the greatest problems.

COMPLEMENTARY AND ALTERNATIVE THERAPIES

Many people with MS—perhaps up to 75 percent—seek to improve their health by approaches considered outside traditional or mainstream Western medicine (National Center for Complementary and Alternative Medicine, 2009). (The word Western is used here to represent standard European and

American medical practices, such as the disease-modifying medications discussed above.) Some approaches, such as certain herbs and acupuncture, are core practices in China, Japan, Korea, and other countries in the Far East. Collectively, these methods are called complementary and alternative therapies: complementary when used in combination with traditional Western medicine, and alternative when used instead of traditional Western treatments. People with MS have tried numerous different approaches, including the following:

- Herbs and dietary supplements
- Stress management techniques, including meditation, yoga, and tai chi
- Biofeedback: a technique aiming to allow individuals to control unconscious bodily processes (such as heartbeats) by making the processes apparent to the senses (such as by an oscilloscope) and then teaching persons how to manipulate these bodily functions
- Massage and other types of bodywork, including the Alexander technique (movement therapy that focuses on posture and other body movements, to reduce muscle strain and tension), Rolfing or Aston variations (deep pressure applied to realign tissues covering muscles and internal organs), Shiatsu (a Japanese technique aimed at increasing circulation and restoring energy balance to the body), and various massage approaches (such as kneading, compression, quick tapping movements of the hands, and vibration)
- Chiropractic: a technique that aims to improve functioning and reduce pain by aligning and adjusting the vertebral column, and sometimes the pelvis and other joints; chiropractors apply pressure with their hands to patients to produce this realignment of the vertebrae and release pressure on nerves
- Acupuncture: a group of techniques, which originated in China and other Asian countries thousands of years ago and involve stimulating certain anatomical points on the body using various methods; in the best-known acupuncture technique, practitioners insert thin, solid, metal needles through the patient's skin at specified points on the body called meridians, aiming to unlock the flow of vital energy

Unlike traditional Western medications, which are tested and regulated by the U.S. Food and Drug Administration to ensure their safety and effectiveness, complementary and alternative therapies are not subject to this scrutiny. This raises concern about safety, especially of therapies involving pills or dietary products. Many herbs and dietary supplements are marketed as so-called natural products, making them sound safe and low risk. However, ingesting almost any compound can carry some level of risk, for example, an allergic reaction or an interaction with a prescription medication. Manufacturers of these products do not receive the same oversight and inspections as do standard drug makers. This raises questions about the safety, dosage strength, and purity of these products.

Because MS symptoms often wax and wane, it is generally difficult for individual patients to know whether improving—or worsening—symptoms resulted from a treatment or from their underlying disease course. As noted above, medications undergo rigorous research studies, sometimes comparing drugs with placebos (sugar pills) across lots of patients. Few complementary or alternative therapies have undergone such research among persons with MS. Therefore, individual patients should be cautious about using complementary or alternative therapies that could pose risks, such as herbal preparations or dietary supplements. People should stay alert for potential side effects of compounds they ingest.

Over recent years, various claims of dramatic improvements from alternative treatments for MS have generated newspaper headlines, only to be disproved by systematic research. One favorite claim, which periodically resurfaces, is that bee venom treats MS. Bee venom therapy typically involves sticking arms or other body parts into cages full of buzzing bees, aiming to be stung. A clinical study of bee venom, however, found no benefit. Another widely circulated claim was that the amalgam of older dental fillings, which contained mercury, causes or worsens MS. This assertion led to many people having their dental fillings removed and replaced with newer compounds. While heavy metals, such as mercury, can damage the nervous system, the pathological process of this damage is different from that observed in MS. Therefore, no logical connection exists between older dental fillings and MS.

One area that is undergoing active research is whether the active ingredient of marijuana (Cannabis sativa, a type of hemp plant) might benefit persons with MS. In particular, some assert that cannabis helps control MS pain and spasticity. Doing a placebo-controlled study of marijuana is difficult. Persons taking the actual marijuana compound become high (experience the mind-altering effects of the drug), while those using any placebo compound would not. Nonetheless, the active ingredient in marijuana (tetrahydrocannabinol) is undergoing testing for spasticity, tremor, and balance in MS. To date, results are mixed. Some studies have shown short-lasting benefits (several hours), while others have found the compound worsens the problem (balance and tremor). Persons have also reported side effects from taking tetrahydrocannabinol, including weakness, mental fogginess, dry mouth, dizziness, and worsened coordination. Further research may produce additional findings about whether tetrahydrocannabinol benefits persons with MS.

MS is a lifelong disease, with few treatment options for many persons. Therefore, persons should be encouraged and supported in doing activities that might make them feel better, in general, rather than aiming specifically to treat their MS. For instance, stress management programs, meditation, yoga, tai chi, exercises, biofeedback, and similar efforts might improve persons' overall sense of health and well being. An additional benefit is that persons might feel in better control of their health. However, some approaches that might seem benign (not dangerous) can carry risks for persons with MS. For example, vigorous massage might be harmful for persons with osteoporosis (thin bones) related to long-standing MS or lengthy glucocorticoid therapy. German massage techniques, which link hand massages with hot baths, may drain strength from persons with heat sensitivity.

Lester Goodall, introduced in Chapter 3, has found something that works for him. According to Mr. Goodall, he is "still exploring mind over matter. They say the immune system is controlled by the brain. I try to find that inner sweet spot. My wife thinks I'm crazy. I do things just for the theatrics, to force feeling. I put my hands out like this," Lester holds both hands out straight in front of him,

and I try to communicate with my immune system. I say two things: "heal and protect." It can't cure me, but heal and protect. Sometimes I think it works. Other times I'm not sure. I can't quantitate it, but there's times when I think I feel better. That keeps me doing it when I'm feeling real bad. That's when I revert back to it: heal and protect.

7

Disability and Rehabilitation Therapies

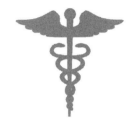

S ally Ann Jones has a new problem. "Four months ago, I fell. It has taken me three months, but now I can stand. And I can move one foot, easily —well, not actually easily, but I can move it. Now I'm working on the other foot, but it's slow."

The problem is that, without being able to stand securely and pivot her body, Sally Ann Jones can no longer do many basic maneuvers safely. For instance, she cannot transfer easily from her scooter wheelchair to her bed, and she cannot get onto and off of the toilet. Mrs. Jones has seen her neurologist repeatedly since she fell, asking him for advice about her pivoting problem.

> My doctor says there are no medicines he can give me—he says there's nothing he can do. He says that, maybe if I keep myself going long enough, there will be a major discovery, a new drug for MS that will help. But how can I get along, day in and day out, if I can't stand and pivot?

What Mrs. Jones needs now is someone skilled in helping her think through how she can safely perform the basic physical movements essential to everyday life, as well as training her to avoid falling in the future. Perhaps with exercise Mrs. Jones might be able to strengthen her leg muscles sufficiently so that she can stand securely long enough to pivot from one seat to another. If not, maybe an expert can suggest changes within her home that would improve her safety, such as positioning grab bars near her toilet or ensuring her bed and wheelchair seat are approximately the same height. What Mrs. Jones needs is a skilled rehabilitation specialist.

None of the medications discussed in Chapter 6 can improve the physical functioning of persons with MS, such as the ability to walk, stand, and use their hands. Although these drugs may shorten MS flares or slow the progression of the disease for some persons and for some period of time, none of them can reduce or eliminate disability. Rehabilitation therapy is the best treatment for meeting those goals.

Broadly defined, rehabilitation involves exercises, assistive technologies, or other therapies that help patients either to improve their functional abilities or to compensate effectively for permanent functional deficits. Rehabilitation specialists aim to assist persons with disabilities caused by diseases, injuries, congenital conditions, or other reasons to either regain functioning or develop strategies to live with impairments as comfortably and safely as possible. For persons disabled by MS, rehabilitation professionals offer a range of services that might prove to be valuable, such as specific exercises to maintain strength and balance, advice and training concerning mobility aids, and modifications to homes and workplaces to improve safety and accessibility.

Chapters 7, 8, and 9 examine the implications of MS-related disability from various different perspectives. Chapter 8 explores mobility aids, the most common type of assistive technology used by persons with MS. Chapter 9 looks at the services and approaches persons disabled by MS need to live independently, comfortably, safely, and productively in their homes and communities. This chapter looks at the role of rehabilitation therapy in MS. Chapter 7 starts by discussing how neurologists assess MS disability. The chapter then describes the history of rehabilitation and the major categories of rehabilitation professionals who treat persons with MS. Chapter 7 concludes by examining rehabilitation treatments frequently provided to persons with MS.

EVALUATING DISABILITY IN MS

The diagnosis of MS is made primarily through the clinical history and physical examination, although such tests as MRI scans assist the diagnostic process (see Chapter 5). Similarly, evaluation of disability—the extent of impaired functioning, such as difficulties walking, standing, using hands and fingers, and swallowing and problems with memory and abstract reasoning—involves taking histories and examining patients. One challenge in evaluating disability during a single office visit is that patients' functioning can vary from day to day and from hour to hour within a single day. If patients become overheated while traveling to the neurologist's office on a hot summer day, they may appear more impaired than usual. Thus, before examining patients, physicians should first ask them about the full range of problems described in Chapter 5. Questions must seek to determine the time course of the person's impairments: whether patients feel their functioning has been generally stable (unchanged) or whether their symptoms are worsening or improving, rapidly or slowly.

Chapter 5 describes approaches neurologists use to evaluate various MS symptoms and functional status, such as muscle strength, coordination, and cognitive processes. Neurologists, physical therapists, and other clinicians have devised various scales or measures to track the disability of persons with MS. Examples include the Expanded Disability Status Scale (EDSS, used widely by American neurologists), the MS Functional Composite, the MS Fatigue Impact Scale, and the Guy's Neurological Disability Scale, named after the famous Guy's Hospital located across the River Thames from the Tower of London in London, United Kingdom.

Some scales concentrate on specific aspects of patients' functioning. The EDSS focuses largely (although not exclusively) on patients' ability to walk, grading persons on a 0 to 10 scale (0 indicates normal neurological examination, while 10 represents death caused by MS). The MS Functional Composite includes a 25-foot walking test. In contrast, the Guy's Neurological Disability Scale grades each of 12 functional domains on a six-point scale, as follows:

0   Normal status
1   Symptoms causing no disability
2   Mild disability—not requiring help from others
3   Moderate disability—requiring help from others
4   Severe disability—almost total loss of function
5   Total loss of function—maximum help required

The 12 functional domains assessed by the Guy's Neurological Disability Scale are (1) cognitive disability, (2) mood disability, (3) visual disability, (4) speech and communication disability, (5) swallowing disability, (6) upper limb disability, (7) lower limb disability, (8) bladder disability, (9) bowel disability, (10) sexual disabilities, (11) fatigue, and (12) other disabilities. The Guy's Neurological Disability Scale specifies the various functional abilities that define the six functional levels for each domain, such as the following for lower limb disability (note that the British refer to canes as sticks and to walkers as frames):

0   Walking is not affected
1   Walking is affected but patient is able to walk independently

2   Usually uses unilateral support (single stick or crutch, one arm) to walk outdoors, but walks independently indoors
3   Usually uses bilateral support (two sticks or crutches, frame, or two arms) to walk outdoors, or unilateral support (single stick or crutch, or one arm) to walk indoors
4   Usually uses a wheelchair to travel outdoors, or bilateral support (two sticks or crutches, frame, or two arms) to walk indoors
5   Usually uses a wheelchair indoors (McDonald and Compston, 2005, 293)

The advantage of using a detailed scale such as the Guy's Neurological Disability Scale is that it forces clinicians to consider the full range of body systems and functions affected by MS. This comprehensive evaluation includes domains that might otherwise be neglected, such as mood problems, fatigue, bladder and bowel problems, and sexual dysfunction. Carefully quantifying disability during office visits over months and years allows neurologists to track the time course of functional impairments, which provides guidance about the patient's prognosis or future experiences with MS.

EDSS, Guy's Neurological Disability Scale, and other disability assessment scales were designed for neurologists to use to evaluate patients. Equally important, however, are scales created for patients to systematically report how MS affects their functioning. Research suggests that some doctors have difficulty accurately assessing patients' functional status, especially since doctors rarely visit patients in their homes to see how they do in environments that are comfortable and familiar to them. Instead, neurologists typically see patients only in the hospital or during office visits, which can be stressful and tiring to patients. Thus, the views of neurologists and patients about patients' functional abilities can differ.

Several questionnaires are available for persons with MS to evaluate their own functioning, including the Multiple Sclerosis Impact Scale, which has 29 questions; the Functional Assessment of Multiple Sclerosis scale, with 44 questions; the Quality of Life Questionnaire for Multiple Sclerosis, with 24 questions; the MS Self-Care Activities of Daily Living Scale, with 15 questions; and a version of the EDSS for patients to answer themselves. As an example about how these questionnaires work, the Multiple Sclerosis Impact Scale asks patients to rate the impact of 29 items during the past two weeks on the following scale (McDonald and Compston, 2005, 295):

Not at all
A little
Moderately

Quite a bit

Extremely

Examples of the 29 items include the following:

- Problems with balance
- Being clumsy
- Difficulties using hands for everyday tasks
- Problems using transportation (e.g., car, bus, train, taxi, etc.)
- Difficulty doing things spontaneously, such as going out on the spur of the moment
- Needing to go to the toilet urgently
- Problems sleeping
- Feeling mentally fatigued
- Feeling irritable, impatient, or short-tempered
- Lack of confidence
- Feeling depressed

To produce an MS impact score, the ratings by patients on each of the 29 items are simply added. Higher scores indicate that MS has a greater impact on patients' daily life than do lower scores. By reviewing how persons rate their own functioning, neurologists can get insight into their patients' perceptions of how MS affects day-to-day activities and their quality of life.

Given the complexities of MS symptoms and disability evaluations, it is tempting to seek straightforward tests, such as MRI scans, to provide objective measures of overall MS disability or functional impairments. As depicted in Figure 5.3, MRI scans of the brains and spinal cords of persons with MS show plaques or areas of myelin destruction caused by the disease process. MRI imaging techniques can quantify the so-called lesion load, the volume of tissue consumed by MS plaques. Perhaps this MRI-detected lesion load relates directly to the extent of MS disability.

Studies have shown, however, that the lesion load, as determined by MRI scan (even with gadolinium enhancement), bears little relationship to the level of disability patients exhibit (Olek, 2008c). Lesions—including large plaques—detected on MRI scan may not produce specific impairments noticed by patients or apparent on physical examinations. Similarly, MRI scans may not pick up plaques corresponding to the area of the brain or spinal cord implicated by a specific functional impairment. Persons with relatively small lesion loads on MRI scans may have profound disability and extensive impairments, while those with large lesion loads may display few impairments. Scientists are still trying to understand completely the source of discrepancies between patients' impairments and clinical symptoms and MRI scan results.

OVERVIEW OF REHABILITATION PROFESSIONS

The overall goal of rehabilitation therapies is to restore or maintain patients' functional abilities or—if this is not possible—to minimize functional losses. If persons become unable to function in particular domains, such as mobility, rehabilitation therapists help devise ways to compensate for those losses. The field of rehabilitation encompasses a half dozen distinct professions, including a specialty of medicine (physical medicine and rehabilitation [PM&R], also known as physiatry) and several disciplines called collectively the allied health professions, including physical therapy, occupational therapy, recreational therapy, and speech-language pathology.

Although these various rehabilitation professionals treat persons of all ages, ranging from earliest childhood to late in life, various chronic conditions related to aging demand rehabilitation services most frequently. Persons with arthritis, back or spine problems, heart disease, stroke, chronic lung disease, and diabetes often seek rehabilitation services to help them improve or maintain their physical functioning. Within the rehabilitation professions, there are specialists who concentrate on very specific areas, such as addressing the needs of athletes or musicians (for example, violin players having trouble with their arms or fingers).

Although persons with MS use a variety of different types of rehabilitation services, they most commonly see physical or occupational therapists or PM&R physicians (also called physiatrists). Often, patients see all three types of professionals, each working with the person as members of a multidisciplinary team to address specific concerns. This section starts by reviewing the history of rehabilitation therapy. Then it briefly describes each of these three major rehabilitation fields.

History of the Rehabilitation Professions

All three professions—physical therapy, occupational therapy, and physiatry (PM&R)—emerged from efforts following World War I to rehabilitate injured veterans. From the onset, rehabilitation therapy for wounded military personnel typically involved multidisciplinary teams (professionals from different disciplines or fields working together) to treat individual patients. In these teams, representatives of the three fields—physical and occupational therapists and doctors, in those early days represented primarily by orthopedic surgeons—played fundamentally different roles on these teams.

In early 1918, as World War I was ending, the Army Orthopedic Service at Walter Reed Hospital outside Washington, D.C., established a nascent rehabilitation service using civilian women as so-called physiotherapists (physical therapists) and occupational therapists. Both groups were known by the general title of reconstruction aides. Although the military initially planned to hire men for these positions, personnel shortages forced them to employ women to treat injured World War I veterans.

Physical therapy reconstruction aides received six weeks of medically oriented training, while occupational therapy aides initially did not. Physical therapy reconstruction aides worked closely with doctors to improve specific aspects of the physical functioning of injured servicemen, such as strengthening particular muscles or muscle groups. Thus, the evaluation and treatment approach of physical therapists became closely allied with approaches physicians used to evaluate and address patients' needs. Physical therapists evaluated and quantified the ability of various muscles, joints, and body structures to move and function.

In contrast, post–World War I occupational therapy aides concentrated primarily on vocational reeducation: training injured veterans in skills related to jobs or occupations and returning to the workforce. Using occupation or job skills to promote or restore health has precedents reaching back to ancient Egypt, Greece, and Rome, which celebrated productive activity alongside art, music, dance, and exercise as pathways to health. Centuries later, the Arts and Crafts movement, imported from England where it began in the 1850s, urged persons to transcend daily anxieties by weaving baskets, building furniture, shaping clay pots, and carving wooden ornaments, among other productive pursuits. After World War I, occupational therapy aides at Walter Reed Hospital initially received little training. Medical authorities saw their work as diverting the minds of injured soldiers away from depression and grief. They taught knitting, basket weaving, raffia work, bead work, rug making, toy and ornament making, and crocheting (Hoover, 1996). But within several years, occupational therapy aides received more formal training focused on vocational rehabilitation, with curricula including anatomy, kinesiology, physiology, and psychology. Occupational therapists also became experts in training wounded veterans to use prostheses (primarily artificial arms and hands) and orthotics (splints).

While the American Occupational Therapy Association and American Physical Therapy Association were established in 1917 and 1921, respectively, the American Congress of Rehabilitation Medicine was founded only in 1933 and the PM&R Academy in 1938. In the early twentieth century, orthopedists—surgeons who specialize in treating bones and attached soft tissues (such as tendons, ligaments, and muscles)—were denigrated as mere sawbones.

Treating wounded World War I soldiers gave orthopedists credibility and catalyzed early medical rehabilitation efforts, primarily designing prosthetics (artificial limbs) and orthotics to improve mobility of injured veterans.

Between World War I and World War II, rehabilitation physicians gained attention for their work with survivors of polio, often a profoundly debilitating disease that was epidemic in the United States. With World War II and the massive influx of seriously wounded veterans, physicians extended their goals to comprehensive restoration of physical, mental, emotional, vocational, and social abilities. Even scientists designing new prosthetic limbs—the trademark technology of rehabilitation specialists confronting numerous veterans with limbs amputated by massive war injuries—emphasized restoring the whole person, not just the arms and legs.

Physical Therapy

The goals of physical therapy are as follows:

- To restore patients' physical functioning to its original or baseline level following an acute event, such as an injury or illness; or,
- If restoring physical function is not possible because of patients' underlying diseases or conditions, to maximize patients' functional abilities and prevent future declines.

Physical therapists evaluate and measure patients' muscle strength, range of motion (extent to which limbs or extremities can move around joints), balance, coordination, posture, fatigue, pain, and other physical functional abilities. After this evaluation, physical therapists generally aim to work collaboratively with patients to develop treatment plans that meet patients' needs and personal circumstances for maximizing their physical functioning.

Physical therapy treatments generally include various exercises, including exercises to strengthen muscles, extend or maintain range of motion, reduce spasticity, keep muscles and joints flexible, and improve endurance. Physical therapists also train patients on strategies to prevent or minimize the risk of falls. In addition, physical therapists evaluate patients for mobility aids, such as canes, walkers, or wheelchairs (see Chapter 8), and teach patients how to use this equipment. Physical therapists work in hospitals, outpatient clinics, and private offices, and some also visit patients' homes to conduct evaluations and provide treatments.

Becoming a physical therapist requires considerable training, including coursework in anatomy, biology, human physiology, and biomechanics. Students then begin working with patients in outpatient offices, clinics, and hospitals, under close supervision of their instructors. To be eligible to practice physical therapy, students must obtain a master's degree (two years of graduate training) or doctoral degree (three years of graduate training). According to the American Physical Therapy Association (www.apta.org), the profession aims that by 2020 all physical therapists will hold doctoral degrees. The APTA Web site indicates that 210 accredited physical therapy training programs are available in the United States.

States require physical therapists to pass a national licensure examination and obtain a license before they can practice. According to the federal Bureau of Labor Statistics *Occupational Outlook Handbook, 2008–09 Edition* (U.S. Department of Labor, 2008), in 2006 there were 173,000 physical therapy jobs in the United States. Because of the aging population—and growing numbers of elderly individuals with chronic conditions (such as arthritis, heart disease, and stroke) that require physical therapy services—the demand for physical therapists is expected to increase by 27 percent from 2006 to 2016.

Occupational Therapy

The ultimate goal of occupational therapy is to assist persons with disabilities to live safely and independently in their homes and communities and to participate fully in daily activities, such as employment and leisure pursuits. According to the American Occupational Therapy Association, Inc. (www.aota.org), occupational therapists aim to help patients live better with illness and disability. Occupational therapy treatment focuses on training or retraining patients in performing various basic skills required in daily life, involving not only physical activities (such as dressing and bathing) but also cognitive and mental functions (such as memory and reasoning skills). An occupational therapist might train patients in manual dexterity skills, such as fastening clothing (e.g., buttoning shirts or tying shoe laces) or in managing short-term memory loss (e.g., training in making lists or reminder strategies).

Occupational therapists can recommend various types of equipment or changes to homes to allow patients to function more easily and safely in their environments. This could include mobility aids (see Chapter 8), devices to help with dressing (such as button hooks, which pull buttons through button holes when patients' fingers cannot manage that task), and cooking utensils that are easier and safer to manage than standard utensils. Occupational therapists therefore frequently perform home evaluations, observing patients as they perform daily tasks within their own environments and assessing homes for threats to safety (such as electrical cords that could trip patients or cooking appliances that pose risks) or barriers to mobility (such as stairs or narrow doorways).

Some occupational therapists focus specifically on patients' driving skills, recommending adaptive equipment (such as hand controls for acceleration and braking) to allow patients to continue driving safely.

To become an occupational therapist, students must obtain either a master's or doctoral degree from an accredited program. In 2007, 124 institutions offered master's programs, and 66 provided combined bachelor's and master's degrees in the United States. Class work includes basic biology, human anatomy and physiology, and social sciences. Students must also perform at least six months of fieldwork or internships, under supervision of instructors.

States require that persons pass a national examination before they can be licensed to practice occupational therapy. In 2006, there were 99,000 occupational therapy jobs in the United States (U.S. Department of Labor, 2008). Employment of occupational therapists is expected to grow by 23 percent between 2006 and 2016, spurred by increasing numbers of elderly individuals who require their services.

Physical Medicine and Rehabilitation

Physical medicine and rehabilitation is a field of medicine. As noted above, PM&R physicians are also called physiatrists (generally pronounced fizz-eye'-ah-trests, although different pronunciations are in use). The Advisory Board for Medical Specialties accepted PM&R as a specialty in 1947. After graduating from medical school, physicians complete a one-year internship in medicine or other general field before entering a three-year PM&R training program. Some physiatrists seek additional fellowship training to specialize in specific areas, such as musculoskeletal conditions, spinal cord injury, traumatic brain injury, sports medicine, or pediatric PM&R. According to the American Academy of Physical Medicine and Rehabilitation (www.aapmr.org), more than 7,500 physiatrists currently practice in the United States.

Physiatrists aim to maximize patients' physical functioning and decrease bodily pain without surgery. They are experts in the functioning of muscles, nerves, joints, and bones, and they rely largely upon clinical histories, physical examinations, and noninvasive tests (such as MRI and other imaging studies, evoked potentials [see Chapter 5], and nerve conduction studies) to evaluate patients. After physiatrists diagnose and evaluate patients, they design treatment plans to address patients' individual goals. Some plans involve assisting patients in managing their own conditions, while others involve other rehabilitation professionals (such as physical and occupational therapists) in teams coordinated by the physiatrist.

REHABILITATION SERVICES FOR MS

Nowadays, rehabilitation typically involves a collaboration between patients and rehabilitation professionals, with patients playing an active role in setting targets or goals and joining with the rehabilitation experts in designing a program to achieve those goals (Kraft and Cui, 2005; Stevenson and Playford, 2007). Goals of rehabilitation therapy for persons with MS vary depending on individual preferences and circumstances. These goals will also vary by extent of functional impairments and disability. Core members of the professional team may include practitioners from the following:

- Neurology
- PM&R, preferably a physiatrist expert in MS
- Physical therapy
- Occupational therapy

Depending on the individual patient's needs, other team members might include a

- MS nurse specialist, to work alongside physicians in assessing patients' needs, such as monitoring their overall ability to perform daily activities (bathing, dressing, toileting, preparing meals, etc.), bladder and bowel functioning, skin integrity (looking for possible pressure ulcers caused by immobility), and psychological concerns
- Speech and language pathologist if the patient has trouble with speech or swallowing; this clinician can help patients learn safe swallowing techniques so that they can eat as normally as possible
- Psychologist, if the patient has problems relating to mood, emotional functioning, or cognitive abilities
- Urologist or other professional expert in bladder and bowel functioning, if the patient has problems with incontinence, constipation, or difficulty voiding urine
- Social worker, to assist with connecting patients to community services, handling insurance or financial issues, or addressing family and social support concerns
- Dietician, if diet or healthy eating issues are present
- Expert in assistive technology or devices, such as orthotics (splints) and mobility aids (see Chapter 8)

Coordinating contributions from these diverse professionals is essential. Primary care physicians, who typically have limited training in neurology, may feel they do not have sufficient clinical expertise to lead the team. Specialized centers that care specifically for persons with MS have been developed to provide this team-based care, often led by nurse experts or other individuals trained in overseeing multidisciplinary care. Organized in 1986, the Consortium of Multiple Sclerosis Centers (CMSC) represents these specialized programs worldwide and can provide information about the location of these centers in the United States (www.mscare.org/cmsc/home.html). These services are located primarily in large cities, so many persons with MS may not have a specialized MS center nearby.

Depending on the individual needs, goals, and preferences of MS patients, MS rehabilitation therapy could involve a range of different activities. Several issues are described below, but individual treatment plans can involve numerous other types of interventions, customized for each individual patient. Chapter 8 discusses essential tools for restoring mobility to persons who can no longer walk independently: ambulation aids and wheeled mobility aids.

Spasticity

Spasticity occurs when muscles continually contract, causing stiffness and tightness. Increased muscle tone and clonus (a series of rapid muscle contractions) can interfere with walking and other physical activities. When spasticity is severe, it can cause pain and uncontrollable muscle spasms. Constant spasticity can also shrink and shorten muscles. Although medications such as baclofen can treat spasticity, drugs frequently have side effects that can also prove to be troublesome. In particular, drugs for treating spasticity can cause fatigue, weakness, and drowsiness.

Frequent stretching exercises offer the most basic and fundamental treatment for spasticity. Therapists should design these exercises so that different muscle groups do not fight each other but instead function in complementary ways, to reduce painful tightness and tension. Range of motion exercises aim to ensure that muscles do not tighten or stiffen around joints, reducing persons' abilities to move, rotate, and flex their limbs. Ideally, persons should do exercises to counteract spasticity every few hours throughout the day.

Weakness and Exercise

Persons without neurological diseases typically exercise to build muscle strength. For persons weakened by MS, exercise will not restore muscle strength. Nevertheless, exercise can provide important benefits in terms of improving strength or slowing its decline. Exercise also has significant psychological advantages, improving mood, a person's sense of control, and quality of life.

Progressive resistance exercises, in which the workload of muscles is increased by increments (such as by adding increasing amounts of weight to a weight-lifting regimen), can help strengthen muscles. Physiatrists and physical therapists work with patients to design and oversee an exercise program, which patients can perform in their homes, physical fitness centers, or other locations. Some patients may prefer home-based exercise programs, since traveling to fitness centers may tire them, making them less able to exercise and defeating the purpose of the journey. Different patients, however, may prefer exercising around other people, finding that camaraderie motivates them to try harder and keep going. Customizing exercise programs for each individual must take these personal preferences into account.

Historically, physicians worried that patients with MS who exercised would become overheated and fatigued, thus defeating the purpose of exercise. One potential solution involves so-called cooling, which lowers the temperatures of persons heated during exercise. Exercising in a cool pool, where the water temperature is less than 85 degrees Fahrenheit, also counteracts heat intolerance and offers the additional benefit of water's buoyancy.

People like the notion that exercises target specific muscles—it makes sense. "I go to a wonderful physical therapist," said Professor Margaret Freemont, who had had MS for decades (Iezzoni, 2003). "Her name is Anna. She explains why you do things, what you're trying to do with certain exercises." Professor Freemont loves doing her exercises. "I'm very motivated; I'm a very compliant patient. Anna and I are working on my posture, standing erect, recruiting muscles that will make me walk better. I will be more alert. I will stand up straighter." She is certain that straightening her posture will improve her ability to walk.

Foot Drop

Certain muscles are especially weak in MS and difficult to strengthen through exercises. Rehabilitation teams must therefore consider other measures to preserve functioning. In particular, among the weakest muscles in persons with MS are those muscles in and around the ankle that cause the foot to flex upward and lift off the ground when patients walk. Because of this weakness, persons experience so-called foot drop—when the leg swings forward as patients walk, the drooping foot drags the ground, stubbing toes, and sometimes causing tripping and dangerous falls. Foot drop gets worse as persons become more fatigued, exacerbating risks of falling.

While persons can try exercise to strengthen ankle muscles, the most direct treatment is generally a plastic ankle-foot orthotic (AFO)—a splint or brace made from plastic or composite materials, which is inserted in the person's shoe and keeps the foot from bending downward and dropping during gait. AFOs come in two basic styles, rigid or articulated (AFOs with hinges, which allow some movement). Certain AFOs produce spring-like actions, conveying energy as the toes lift from the ground while stabilizing the ankle. Devising the best AFO for individual patients requires careful physical evaluation by a physiatrist or other skilled rehabilitation professional, to assess muscle strength, spasticity, and other biomechanical factors that contribute to foot drop. Then, a skilled orthotist must produce and adjust the AFO to fit each individual patient.

For persons with mild leg weakness, in whom foot drop is the major problem, new functional electrical stimulation (FES) devices are showing great promise in improving gait. To counteract foot drop, FES involves positioning a small, battery-powered device below the knee on the affected leg. During the swing phase of the gait cycle, the device emits an electrical signal that stimulates the nerve that controls the muscles and causes the foot to flex upward. The low-level FES electrical signal does not shock or cause pain. Instead it prompts the muscle contractions that allow virtually normal walking, with appropriate upward flexion of the foot as its leg swings forward. With FES, persons with MS whose only mobility problem involves foot drop can walk safely, no longer afraid of falls from a drooping foot.

Home Evaluations and Activities of Daily Living

Marsha is an occupational therapist who visits patients in their homes (Iezzoni, 2003). She evaluates how patients do their daily activities within their home, and then she works with patients to find strategies to make these activities easier, safer, less stressful, and less fatiguing. Marsha described a patient with MS who "was sleeping on the floor because she could not get up. When she went to do something, she fell. She felt it was just easier to spend her life crawling around her floor, and she did it for a long time."

To assist the patient, Marsha thought of various different strategies, ranging from grab bars, to wheelchairs, to repositioning furniture, to finding alternative ways for the woman to perform routine activities. All the while, the woman expressed her reluctance to recognize her physical limitations and the likelihood of progression. Marsha therefore needed to consider psychological factors and the emotional consequences of her strategies and suggestions to the patient.

"Occupational therapy focuses nowadays on the importance of client-centered goals," Marsha observed, "goals that clients help make. They're able to assess the outcome so they can actually see how they're doing. They really own their goal. Patients are part of the process from the first interaction."

Another home-based occupational therapist Jennifer agreed, especially when patients need extensive education.

Sometimes you have to teach people they need to conserve their energy but they also need to exercise. I teach them energy conservation and pacing. I'm trying to work on this with an MS patient right now. She doesn't understand why she just can't do things the way she's always done them. I'm doing a lot of teaching on why she needs to conserve her energy. She shouldn't make all these trips back and forth across her apartment. She should get everything at once and bring it over. I'm trying to teach her to prioritize and to schedule exercise sessions and rest periods.

"A lot of what we do is encourage people to be as independent as possible," said Marsha.

If they don't start doing something, they'll never be able to do it. I worked with a patient today. In that half hour, she must have said a hundred times, "I don't want to live like this; I don't want to live like this." So I say, "Well, the reason I'm here is to help you to do more for yourself. You need to work with me so we can do that."

8

Ambulation Aids and Wheeled Mobility Aids

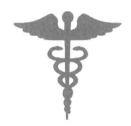

At first, I had no choice about using a cane. While walking home one day during my third year of medical school, my right leg collapsed without warning (Iezzoni, 2003). The fall broke a small bone on the outer margin of my foot—the fifth metatarsal. The fracture was minor, and the pain abated within a week. Nevertheless, to heal the bone, I couldn't put weight on the foot. I therefore needed to use a cane, off-loading my weight onto the cane rather than my right leg. Afterward, the cane became necessary to steady my veering, unbalanced gait.

Using the cane embarrassed me. The continual barrage of eerily identical questions was also annoying: "What happened to you? Did you have a skiing accident?" It was late winter and in Boston, where many enjoy that often-risky sport, so it was logical to ask a young adult using a cane about skiing injuries. But I had never skied in my life, unless you count an unhappy hour in high school. Taking the rope tow up the beginner slope, unsteady on rented skis, I felt an unpleasant choking sensation. The twisting rope tow had latched onto the fringe of the scarf looped around my neck and was progressively strangling me. After they stopped the tow and unwound me, I sat out the rest of the day. I never tried skiing again.

So how do you answer such questions? "No, I didn't have a skiing accident," sounds inadequate, too terse, and unfriendly. Social convention seemed to force me to say more, giving a complete explanation. But I didn't want to. As a third-year medical student, I wanted to hide my MS; it was private, my business alone. In addition, because I was not yet a full-fledged doctor, I felt the issue might affect my interactions with patients. If I mentioned my MS, I reasoned, patients may lose respect for me or might think I sought their sympathy. Burdening them with my illness and shifting the focus to me, even by explaining my cane, was presumptuous. After all, they were the ones who were sick, lying in hospital beds.

Plus, the cane was clunky. When I propped it in a corner while examining or talking to patients, the cane always toppled, falling with a clatter onto the shiny waxed floors. If instead I laid the cane on the floor in those cramped hospital rooms, someone, including me, could trip over it. Girded by these rationalizations, I began stashing (hiding) the cane at the nurse's station or utility room before entering patients' rooms, carefully clutching the doorframe for balance. That way, maybe patients wouldn't notice I had trouble walking.

* * * * *

Mobility aids are always visible, and they are explicitly utilitarian. Unlike the svelte, glossy black walking sticks twirled by dancers in Hollywood musicals and theatrical extravaganzas, real mobility aids aim clearly to support or transport persons. These aids generally do their jobs well, enhancing balance, maximizing safety, easing pain, and helping people get around. Mobility aids can restore independence and conserve energy drained by enervating struggles to walk.

Nevertheless, users of mobility aids openly admit—both to themselves and to the outside world—their difficulty walking and need for mechanical assistance. Walking short-term with canes or crutches after an athletic accident or other injury is one thing. Presumably, all will heal, and the canes or crutches will vanish into a closet to gather dust and be forgotten. But long-term, mobility aids carry not only weight, quite literally, but also a hefty symbolism. For someone with MS, canes typically shout out the beginning of a functional decline, that slippery downhill slope toward a wheelchair.

Not surprisingly, therefore, many people with progressive disabling conditions such as MS express tremendous ambivalence about using mobility aids. They try to avoid them as long as possible. But at some point, using equipment to aid mobility simply becomes necessary. People no longer have a choice. When that happens, perhaps paradoxically, people may find the world opens up to them again. For me, starting to use a battery-powered scooter felt like spring after a housebound winter. I could zip around where I pleased, at maximum speed (four to five miles per hour), no longer exhausted and terrified of falling. Why had I waited so long?

Chapter 8 explores these psychological dimensions and also introduces the range of mobility aids that persons with MS might use to get around. The chapter groups mobility aids into two broad types:

- Ambulation aids: canes, crutches, and walkers, used by persons who are still ambulating (walking); and
- Wheeled mobility aids: manual wheelchairs (wheelchairs self-propelled by the user or pushed from behind by a walking person), power wheelchairs (wheelchairs that move as directed by the user and powered by batteries), and battery-powered scooters (which function as wheelchairs and have either three or four small wheels).

Chapter 8 reviews the role of different mobility aids for persons with MS, looking in greater depth at the history of wheelchairs, which have witnessed tremendous technological advances in the last three decades. Sophisticated wheeled mobility aids today can cost many thousands of dollars. Chapter 8 therefore concludes by examining how health insurance covers mobility aids. The chapter starts by examining walking problems among persons with MS and patterns of mobility aid use.

WALKING DIFFICULTIES AMONG PERSONS WITH MS

As described in Chapter 5, persons with MS can experience disabling impairments that range, quite literally, from head to toe. Some persons report that problems with vision are their biggest difficulty, while others highlight bladder or bowel incontinence, and yet others underscore fatigue. Every patient has his or her own unique story about the most troubling impairments caused by MS.

As indicated in Table 5.1, walking problems are the second most commonly reported symptom of MS, following fatigue. But difficulty walking is generally the MS impairment that is most visible to the outside world. Difficulties walking inevitably interfere with performing daily activities and doing other things that people enjoy. Thus, walking difficulties can contribute to depression and sadness, worsening quality of life. Walking difficulties also cause falls, with possibly dangerous injuries. Incontinence is even more incapacitating when walking troubles impede speedy transit to the toilet. Therefore, walking impairments can have ripple effects beyond the immediate concern about getting from point A to point B.

There are no precise estimates of how many persons with MS require mobility aids at some point over their lifetimes. It is generally believed that about one-third of persons with MS will need at least a unilateral cane (a single cane or cane on only one side) within 10 years of disease onset (Compston and Coles, 2002). More than 80 percent will require at least a unilateral cane by 30 years after their MS begins. Unlike other conditions, such as spinal cord injury, where specific neurological lesions compromise leg function, many factors can contribute to MS mobility problems, including the following:

- Weakness
- Spasticity: spasms or involuntary contractions of the muscles or muscle fibers
- Ataxia: lack of ability to coordinate voluntary muscle movements
- Imbalance: typically caused by abnormalities in the cerebellum of the brain and related central nervous system tracts
- Clonus: involuntary muscle contractions followed by partial relaxation, resulting in repetitive beating or pulsing movements
- Heat sensitivity
- Fatigue

In 2007, my colleagues and I conducted a telephone survey of 703 persons ages 23 to 67 years old who have MS and lived in homes and apartments (not nursing homes, where some persons severely impaired by MS reside) throughout the United States (Iezzoni, Rao, and Kinkel, 2009). All these people had had MS for at least two years. The survey asked respondents about their mobility problems and use of mobility aids. Almost 68 percent said that their MS had limited their ability to walk in the previous 12 months, and 56 percent reported having fallen in the prior year because of their MS. Among those who reported walking limitations, 82 percent used a mobility aid.

Based on the survey results, Table 8.1 indicates various types of problems reported by survey respondents—this time in the previous two weeks—and how many persons reporting those problems used at least one mobility aid. Needing to concentrate while walking was the most common of the six problems shown in Table 8.1; 84 percent of persons reporting this problem used at least one type of mobility aid. About one-fifth of respondents said that MS had limited a lot their ability to walk, and 97 percent of these persons used at least one mobility aid. These survey results suggest the obvious: that when persons with MS experience mobility problems, they turn to mobility aids for assistance.

Table 8.1

Reports of Specific Mobility Problems in Previous Two Weeks and Use of at Least One Mobility Aid

Mobility Problem Related to MS	Percent with Mobility Problem	Percent Using Mobility Aid[a]
Needs to concentrate while walking	79%	84%
Difficulties standing while doing things	70	87
Increased effort needed to walk	59	87
Has to hold onto furniture, walls, or someone's arm when walking indoors every day	40	95
A lot of balance problems while standing or walking	40	93
MS limits a lot the ability to walk	21	97

[a]Percent who had specific mobility difficulty who reported using any mobility aids.
Adapted from Iezzoni, Rao, and Kinkel, 2009.

MOBILITY AID HIERARCHY

Mobility aids fall into a hierarchy, progressing from low-tech wooden canes with crook handles, to multifooted canes, to crutches, to walkers, to manual wheelchairs and scooters, to sophisticated power wheelchairs. People generally start with the lowest practical option and then work their way up the hierarchy if impairments progress. In our 2007 survey of 703 persons nationwide with MS, 60 percent reported using at least one mobility aid during the previous 12 months. But most of these individuals used multiple types of equipment: 20 percent used two different types of mobility aids, and 27 percent used three or more types of aids (Iezzoni, Rao, and Kinkel, 2009). People use different equipment in different contexts and for different purposes. For example, they might use walkers inside their homes, but scooters when traveling outdoors. Table 8.2 shows the percent of persons using different types of mobility aids.

Over the last three decades, the sophistication, design, and diversity of mobility aids have expanded dramatically, offering consumers wide-ranging options for every taste and requirement. Yet little systematic scientific evidence is available about the technical pros and cons of different mobility aids, such as their safety and biomechanics in routine use. Choice of mobility aids must consider many factors beyond lower extremity functioning, including people's level of fatigue, cognitive status and judgment, vision, vestibular function (which affects balance and vertigo), upper body strength, and physical endurance, as well as their home and community environments.

Table 8.2
Types of Mobility Aids Used in Last Year

	Group of Survey Respondents	
Mobility Aid	All Persons (n = 703)	Persons Using at Least One Mobility Aid (n = 434)
Power wheelchair	30%	37%
Scooter	27	32
Manual wheelchair	53	63
Rolling walker	19	32
Standard walker	6	10
Crutches (one or two)	4	6
Cane (one or two)	34	57

Adapted from Iezzoni, Rao, and Kinkel, 2009.

AMBIVALENCE VERSUS NECESSITY

Dr. Stuart Hartman, a physician who developed MS himself and started using a cane, said that his patients sometimes resist using mobility aids, even something as simple as a cane. "Canes are a sign of everything from failure to a public acknowledgement of disability," said Dr. Hartman.

Patients just don't want to be seen that way. They feel like everybody is looking at them, like they're getting old and that's the final chapter. You try to convince them of the advantages, but people say, "Doc, I just won't use it." A lot of people later discover, hey, that was a good idea, and they like it. They may be able to go farther because they're not as exhausted.

For people with progressive disabling conditions, such as MS, the decision to use mobility aids—especially those at the top of the hierarchy, like a wheelchair—often emerges slowly, borne of practical necessity counterbalanced by visions of the future and sense of self. As walking fails, each person's story differs. Some people are resilient; others despair; most fall in between. People's feelings evolve over time, sometimes reaching a steady state of acceptance, although some do not. In our 2007 survey of 703 people with MS, we found that approximately 45 percent of those who used mobility aids initially resisted getting their device. They cited many reasons for this, including the following among manual wheelchair users:

- 89 percent didn't want to give into their MS by using a wheelchair.
- 85 percent worried about a loss of independence.

- 70 percent worried that their walking would worsen if they used the manual wheelchair.
- 53 percent thought that other people would think they are weak if they use the wheelchair.
- 14 percent worried about losing their jobs if they used a wheelchair.
- 12 percent said a family member objected to them using the wheelchair.

Despite this initial trepidation, often people are surprised by the benefits they experience once they start using mobility aids. Journalist John Hockenberry (1995, 207) had no choice about using a wheelchair after his spinal cord injury:

> It took years of being in a wheelchair before I could be truly amazed by what it could do, and what I could do with it. On a winter night in Chicago, after a light snow, I rolled across a clean stretch of pavement and felt the smooth frictionless glide of the icy surface. I made a tight turn and chanced to look around and back from where I had just come. . . . I saw two beautiful lines etched in the snow. They began as parallel and curved, then they crossed in an effortless knot at the place where my wheelchair turned to look back. My chair had made those lines. The knot was the signature of every turn I had ever made . . . It was the first time I dared to believe that a wheelchair could make something, or even be associated with something, so beautiful.

Psychotherapist Rhonda Olkin (1999, 285), who uses a wheelchair because of polio, argues that acceptance of technologies such as mobility aids requires that they must be seen as enabling activities that would otherwise be difficult or impossible to do without them. Some people take this perspective—the cup half full rather than half empty—more easily than do others. But, as Dr. Olkin wrote, the individual person needs to make the choices. Just because someone has lost the ability to walk does not mean they should lose control over making decisions about their mobility strategies. Although working with rehabilitation professionals to select appropriate equipment is strongly advisable (see Chapter 7), at the end of the day the person with MS has to make the final decision. If a mobility aid does not fit their goals and preferences, the person is unlikely to use or benefit from the equipment.

AMBULATION AIDS

Ambulation aids, such as those depicted in Figure 8.1, fall at the low-tech end of the mobility device continuum. Canes are simple but remarkably useful.

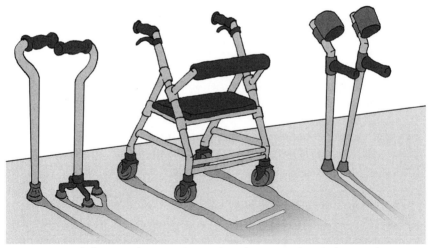

Figure 8.1. Ambulation Aids. Depending on how they are used, ambulation aids improve stability and off-load weight while people walk. This drawing illustrates (from left to right) a single-point cane, three-point cane, rolling walker (with handle-bar brakes and seat), and forearm crutches. [Anil Shukla]

They help off-load weight, as I needed for healing my metatarsal (foot bone) fracture. In MS, canes augment muscle action and provide stability, especially for people with ataxia and imbalance. Canes convey tactile information, which aids in enhancing balance. Canes also improve stability by increasing persons' base of support. If a single (unilateral) cane no longer supplies adequate balancing assistance, persons can use bilateral canes (canes in both their right and left hands).

Oftentimes, people buy canes from drugstores or receive them from family or friends, without getting professional advice or training. Most people get little instruction in proper use of canes, although, as Dr. Hartman notes, "Somebody with a balance disturbance should use a cane differently from someone with arthritis who uses it for weight-bearing." Up to 70 percent of canes are the wrong length, faulty, or damaged, resulting in persons not getting the maximum benefit from their canes. Physical or occupational therapists can assure that persons get the proper equipment and train them to use the ambulation aids to maximum advantage (see Chapter 7).

Although canes are the least sophisticated ambulation aid, several variants are available, differing at their handles and bases (see Figure 8.1). Canes come with crook tops, spade tops, and straight tops; they can have a single, rubber-capped tip or three or four short legs attached to little platforms at their base. Whether these different types of canes provide significantly different types of support is unclear, given limited scientific research concerning this question.

Some believe that multipoint canes (canes with three or four legs) offer superior stability to single-point canes. Furthermore, they like the ability of multipoint canes to stand up on their own, such as next to someone's chair. Others find multipoint canes to be unwieldy and cumbersome. Cane selection largely reflects personal tastes. Again, physical or occupational therapists can provide professional advice to assist patients in making choices that work for them.

Crutches primarily off-load weight rather than improve balance. Therefore, crutches are less adapted to the specific needs of persons with MS mobility problems. As shown in Table 8.2, only 6 percent of persons who use mobility aids employ crutches. Depending on one's upper body strength, underarm crutches can bear up to 100 percent of someone's weight, while forearm crutches (with a cuff and piece fitting under the forearm ending in a handle) can bear 40 to 50 percent. The cuff allows users of forearm crutches to free their hands for activities such as opening doors without removing their crutches. Different styles of crutches offer different benefits for people with weakness in specific arm muscles. Again, choosing the most suitable crutch depends on individual circumstances and would benefit from the skilled assessment of a physical or occupational therapist. As with canes, training and proper fitting maximize their usefulness.

Walkers provide additional stability for people with poor balance and lower extremity weakness. Many types of walkers exist, from standard, rigid models without wheels to collapsible, wheeled walkers with handbrakes, seats, and baskets (see Figure 8.1). As shown in Table 8.2, rolling walkers are much more popular among persons with MS who use mobility aids than are standard models (32 versus 10 percent). As with canes, walkers should be the proper height, and training is essential. Wheeled walkers are dangerous if they roll forward unexpectedly when people lean on them, but they are easy to propel on smooth surfaces, take less energy to use, and require less mental concentration to operate than standard walkers (which must be lifted and moved forward, step by step, as the person advances). In addition, rigid walkers have an institutional appearance, a symbol of debility. Colorful rolling walkers with baskets and seats, in contrast, are practical (for navigating shopping malls, resting when fatigued, and so on) and seem friendlier. People who refuse standard walkers often welcome the rolling version.

Weighing Pros and Cons and Making Choices

Given the range of ambulation aids, persons with MS have a variety of choices (Iezzoni, 2003). Individuals will make decisions about what works best for them based on their personal circumstances and goals. "I needed a cane for balance, for security, for safety," stated Louisa Delarte, an artist, who was concerned about falling. "I thought the cane with four prongs helped more, gives more stability. But I didn't choose it because I was too vain." She felt the four-point cane looked more disabled than the simple single point cane. "I have to be honest, to tell you the truth, I didn't want people staring at me."

Gerald Bernadine, a businessman, also struggled with vanity, but in the end, his fears won out, compelling him to buy his single point cane. "A fractured hip," said Mr. Bernadine, "that's actually my biggest fear. If I fell out here on the pavement and I fractured a hip, that's all I need! That's the reason I started using the cane. It was a safety thing. If I fall, I'm going to be a lot worse off than losing a little vanity. Vanity had prevented me from using the cane."

The off-putting symbolism of ambulation aids is mitigated somewhat by style and color. Specialty shops now offer carved or painted canes that are ornamental as well as practical, and, as noted above, rolling walkers with seats and handlebar brakes come in all sorts of colors and styles. A physical therapist recalled a "young MS patient who was going to a wedding, and she didn't want to take her beaten-up old cane. She's putting on a real fancy dress, and she didn't want to use that icky-looking cane even though it would help her be more mobile walking down the aisle." The patient found a painted cane that met her mobility and aesthetic needs.

"The stigma is heavy duty for some people," observed an experienced occupational therapist.

> They're not going out if they must use a walker or cane, especially young people. They have to go through a process where they feel that it's OK. People look at you, especially if you're young. It's not considered cool, hip, sporty. Thank goodness the equipment is now less nursing home-looking. Like the canes. They're a little bit sporty, and they have all these carved canes.

She feels that rehabilitation therapists must be creative, finding ways to redefine symbols of disability to "feel more comfortable or interesting to patients. Each person needs to find a way to make equipment less of a barrier with other people."

While the vast majority of persons use ambulation aids to assist their walking, people often find one additional benefit—the aids caution strangers to stand clear, to get out of their way. This helps in crowds where people fear being shoved or tripped. These instances offer a contrasting view of the symbolism of ambulation aids: it is good when passersby view persons as disabled and know to keep their distance. Lester Goodall, for instance, cited several motivations for using his cane.

"I have times when I lose my balance," said Mr. Goodall, "that's why I walk with a cane when I'm on the street and when I travel on the public transportation. It gives me something to brace myself." He likes to sit when he's on speeding, swaying subways, but the cars are often crowded during his rush hour morning and evening commutes. Each subway car has seats marked with the wheelchair logo and designated for disabled passengers. Mr. Goodall feels that carrying a cane validates his claim to the reserved seats. "It identifies me to the average person out there. It's a general statement."

* * * * *

The year after medical school graduation, my husband and I went on a brief vacation to London, United Kingdom (Iezzoni, 2003). I still walked with one cane and thought I could get through the trip by using taxis and resting frequently on benches. Most importantly, I had my husband's strong and willing arm. It was early November, and the first day it rained. So we headed to the National Gallery, entering through a little foyer up several stairs. The guard in his navy blue uniform immediately accosted us.

"Do you want a wheelchair?" he asked.

"No, thank you," I answered, somewhat taken aback. Did I look like I needed a wheelchair?

"You might as well take it," he persisted. "You are going to need it sooner or later."

"No, thank you," I said, trying to be firm. "I'll manage." The guard shrugged his shoulders.

This conversation unnerved me. Despite my bravado, was the guard right? I spent that morning searching for benches: I had no choice. My legs held me upright only briefly before threatening collapse. Fortunately, wide sturdy benches are strategically placed throughout the art gallery so I saw the major treasures, albeit from bench distance. But my confidence was rattled.

So passed our trip. I lurched from bench to bench, with some good stretches in between. The unexpected silver lining was our encounters with people. Instead of moving at breakneck speed as do many American tourists, we took our time. Because we were slow, often stationary, people talked to us. The downside was obvious. Every vertical moment, I had to concentrate on remaining erect. I could not look around me, only at my feet below. My husband inched along at a snail's pace, bearing and feeling responsible for a heavy load. Overall, the trip was wonderful—of course, a London vacation would be. But the guard at the National Gallery had been right. I needed a wheelchair.

* * * * *

Several years elapsed before I acceded to the guard's prediction—that I would need a wheelchair sooner or later—and purchased my first scooter-type wheelchair. I raised all the usual objections: using a scooter conceded failure, I would never walk again, my remaining muscle strength would wither, riding was embarrassing, and I didn't want to be seen that way. Plus, having left an awkward girlhood, I relished being tall. In a wheelchair, I would constantly gaze up at the world rather than looking it straight in the eye.

But the countervailing arguments won. My legs carried me shorter and shorter distances, more and more slowly; even brief walks exhausted my strength; I occasionally fell; and I could not travel alone, as my job increasingly demanded. I wanted independence and control over getting around. I desperately wished to walk, but since I couldn't go far, I decided to roll. So I did, and it was terrific! I love my wheelchairs.

* * * * *

WHEELED MOBILITY AIDS

Gerald Bernadine, who had been a high-intensity businessman before coming down with MS (see Chapter 9), and I first talked at a local university where he taught night courses at the school of management. Despite the chilly day, I rode my scooter just over a mile to his office. Mr. Bernadine walked slowly and tentatively into our meeting room, leaning constantly against the wall. With his free hand, he extended a wobbling cane for counterbalance. He collapsed into a chair, collecting himself, before beginning to talk. "I am so exhausted by the end of the day," he said. "My legs feel like they weigh a thousand pounds. I feel like an old man." As I prepared to leave after our conversation, he eyed my scooter. "How did you get over here?" he asked.

"I rode over."

"Really? Can you really go that far on a scooter?"

"Sure," I replied and answered his many questions. He had never thought about a scooter. Several months later, I heard that Mr. Bernadine had bought one, and I wanted to learn more about his decision and experiences. When I rolled over to his office this time, I found Mr. Bernadine zipping around in a bright red scooter, which he called his cart.

"I don't have limits now about where I can go," Mr. Bernadine smiled.

Fortunately, we live in the United States, so there are lots of elevators and ramps, curb cuts, and accessibility. I can shoot around the streets in Boston and do lots of things that I used to dread, like going to the Registry of

Motor Vehicles recently to get my driver's license. You know what that's like with all the lines and waiting—an absolute horror show. No sweat! I just rode up on my little cart, I waited in line with everybody else. I got my license and, zoom, I was out of there.

The other day I taught a three-hour class. No problem. I came in and did all those last minute things before class. I zipped around in my cart. I got everything I needed, and I drove it right into the classroom. I saved all that physical energy. Afterwards, instead of being exhausted—even after a three-hour class—I still had energy.

Mr. Bernadine said that his university colleagues seemed happy that he no longer struggled to get around but warned him humorously to control his impulses. "I need a cow catcher on the front of my cart so I can knock people out of the way! The biggest thing is needing to be careful not to drive too fast, especially in the building. There's a wicked temptation on these long straight-aways to go fast. But I don't want the Dean to get upset, so I'm trying to behave myself with the speed." For Mr. Bernadine, his scooter restored not only his energy and mobility but also his control over important aspects of daily life.

Wheelchair Symbolism and Its Paradox

Perhaps nothing has symbolized frailty, dependence, and loss more completely, definitively, and succinctly than a wheelchair. Words produce images of being lashed in place, immobilized, and constricted.

The ascription of passivity can be seen in language used to describe the relationship between disabled people and their wheelchairs. The phrases *wheelchair bound* or *confined to a wheelchair* are frequently seen in newspapers and magazines, and heard in conversation. . . . The various terms imply that a wheelchair restricts the individual, holds a person prisoner (Linton, 1998, 27).

The threat of needing a wheelchair terrifies persons newly confronting MS. Decades later, philosophy professor S. Kay Toombs (1995, 4) recalled her reaction on being diagnosed with MS at 29 years of age:

Just two days earlier, by strange coincidence, I had read a magazine article about the plight of a young woman with M.S. The photos accompanying the story are still imprinted on my mind. In one, the woman posed coquettishly in a bathing suit with a "Miss Michigan" sash emblazoned across her chest. In the other, she sat dejectedly in a wheelchair, appearing broken and helpless. The author explained she was paralyzed, unable to care for herself . . .

Not surprisingly, on hearing my diagnosis, my first question to the physician was, "Will I end up in a wheelchair?"

One difficulty in outright rejecting wheelchairs as symbols of debility is that they *are* used only when people cannot walk. So one must focus on looking beyond specific physical limitations to the whole person. It is ironic that dependence and lost control are symbolized by wheelchairs, which, by definition, are built around that most enabling of early technologies, the wheel.

Wheels and chairs were probably developed contemporaneously, albeit separately, somewhere in the eastern Mediterranean region around 4000 BC (Kamenetz, 1969). Before then, people sat or squatted on the ground and carried their belongings and other items. Chairs assuredly improved personal comfort, but wheels transformed mankind's sense of space in the world. In various guises, wheels have borne people and their possessions to almost every corner of dry land.

Although canes, crutches, and walkers also symbolize dependence, they carry less stigma than wheelchairs, perhaps because their users retain that upright, bipedal posture which first defined *Homo sapiens*. This distinction is not based on practical functionality. Wheelchairs can be fast, safe, and flexible, as many users will attest. According to author Nancy Mairs (1996, 39), who was diagnosed with MS at age 28, "Certainly I am not mobility impaired; in fact, in my Quickie P100 with two twelve-volt batteries [her power wheelchair], I can shop till you drop at any mall you designate, I promise."

The symbolism of wheelchairs is changing as more wheelchair users participate in public life and appear on the street. Every year at the Boston marathon, for example, the elite wheelers roll off the starting line and finish before the bipedal runners. The Paralympic Games are held following the Summer and Winter Olympics and feature athletes with disabilities within six specific categories, including conditions caused by physical and vision impairments (www.paralympic.org). Wheelchair athletes compete in numerous different and frequently intense Paralympic events, attracting international attention and awe. (The Special Olympics, sometimes confused with the Paralympics, involve athletes with developmental or intellectual disabilities.)

Thus, instead of using metaphors of confinement, language about wheelchair use is also changing. Instead of calling someone "confined to a wheelchair," disability advocates "are more likely to say that someone *uses a wheelchair*. The latter phrase not only indicates the active nature of the user and the positive way that wheelchairs increase mobility and activity but recognizes that people get in and out of wheelchairs for different activities" (Linton, 1998, 27).

Reinventing the Wheel: History of Wheelchairs

Today's wheelchair users go many places, independently and with confidence, because they control equipment designed specifically for their needs. Over the last 30 years, attitudes about wheelchair technology that had persisted for millennia altered dramatically. Throughout history, wheelchairs existed for the convenience of caregivers who needed to move inert human cargo. As Dr. Herman Kamenetz (1969), a physiatrist, recounted in his history of wheelchair technologies, in ancient times, people with limited mobility were transported on litters, carried by slaves, servants, or family members. Even wealthy, walking persons traveled on luxurious palanquins or covered litters, borne on the shoulders of four or more men.

Perhaps the earliest picture of a wheeled chair comes from a Chinese sarcophagus dated about AD 525. By the Middle Ages in Europe, most poor people with impaired mobility were transported short distances in wheelbarrows. Within homes, small wheels were affixed to furniture to roll it around, and people with impaired mobility were placed on this furniture only after it was moved.

Rolling chairs, where both the chair and its occupant move simultaneously, were built during that period but rarely. In 1595, Jehan Lhermite, a Flemish nobleman, crafted a so-called invalid chair for his patron Philip II, King of Spain, who had incapacitating gout (a painful inflammation of the joints caused by uric acid crystals and associated, at that time, with excessive drinking and eating among wealthy men). With its horse hair cushioning, the massive chair optimized the king's comfort, although he could not operate its complicated mechanics himself. According to Lhermite, the king viewed his chair as worth 10 times its weight in gold and silver.

By the early 1700s, some chairs had devices for self-propulsion, including pulleys, cranks, springs, and large wheels. By the 1800s, the most common wheeled chair was the Bath chair, developed in the 1790s by John Dawson at Bath, the English spa and site of Britain's only hot mineral springs. Visited by persons seeking the healing effects of these hot waters, Bath hosted many with impaired mobility who needed assistance getting to and from various bathing and other treatment sites in town. Bath chairs typically had two large wheels in the rear and a smaller wheel in front. While an attendant pushed the chair from behind, its occupant steered using a handle connected to the front wheel.

Wheelchairs first appeared in America to transport wounded soldiers during the Civil War. Primarily made of wood and cane, these heavy chairs had large wooden wheels up front. Later, as bicycles became popular, wheelchairs adopted their lightweight, rubber tires. The 32nd president of the United States, Franklin Delano Roosevelt (1882–1945), who contracted polio at age 39 in 1921 and never walked again, designed his own wheelchair.

> The chair he rode in was a simple device. The standard wheelchair of the day was a cumbersome thing made of wood and wicker . . . impractical for work or travel. So, rather than struggle with such a contraption, Roosevelt had a chair built to his own specifications and design. To the seat and back of a common, straightback kitchen chair he had a sturdy base attached, with two large wheels in front, two small ones in back. . . . Roosevelt seldom sat for long in his wheelchair. Rather, he used it to scoot from his desk chair to a couch, from the couch to the car. He used his chair as a means of movement, not as a place to stay (Gallagher, 1994, 91–92).

In 1918, Herbert A. Everest, a mining engineer, was injured at work and became paraplegic. Dissatisfied with existing wheelchairs, he enlisted mechanical engineer Harry C. Jennings to design sturdier models. Together they founded a company in Los Angeles which, in 1933, manufactured the first folding metal wheelchairs. Their revolutionary design cut the weight of wheelchairs from 90 to 50 pounds (Shapiro, 1994). Their company, Everest & Jennings (E & J), dominated the wheelchair market for the next 50 years. In particular, E & J supplied wheelchairs to hospitals and nursing homes. But E & J failed to notice the growing numbers of new wheelchair users who wanted to live full and active lives, not constrained by unwieldy mobility aids. One dissatisfied consumer was Marilyn Hamilton, who in 1978 had crashed her hang glider into a California mountainside and became paraplegic.

> Hamilton zipped through rehabilitative therapy in three weeks. Most people take at least three months. Then she was impatient with the bulky wheelchair—"a stainless steel dinosaur," she called it—that her physical therapist ordered for her. Hamilton loved sports but the wheelchair was too heavy to get back out on the tennis court. So Hamilton sought out her friends and fellow glider pilots Don Helman and Jim Okamoto. . . . Build me an ultralight wheelchair, Hamilton asked them, out of the aluminum tubing you put in your gliders (Shapiro, 1994, 211).

The resulting wheelchair was sky blue and weighed 26 pounds instead of the standard 50. Hamilton, Helman, and Okamoto went into business, selling so-called Quickie wheelchairs.

> Hamilton's wheelchairs put people—users and those around them—at ease. Instead of chrome, Hamilton's chairs came in a rainbow of hot colors. The customer could personalize a chair in candy apple red, canary yellow, or electric green. . . . "Screaming neon chairs," Hamilton called them. A Quickie chair was fun, refuting the idea that the user was an invalid. (Quickie's biggest competitor today is Invacare, a name that is an abbreviation for "invalid care.") Quickie chair riders were neither sick nor objects of pity. They just got around in a different way. "If you can't stand up," Hamilton likes to say, "stand out" (Shapiro, 1994, 212).

My Quickie manual wheelchair is forest green.

Some give partial credit to Quickie designs for furthering the disability rights movement of the 1980s, described in Chapter 9. Quickie designs expanded the independence of wheelchair users. Even the name Quickie is a lighthearted, double entendre, mocking the assumption that sex life ends when legs stop working.

The market success of Quickie and continuing needs for new technologies (such as a lightweight power wheelchair) attracted many competitors to the wheelchair market. Even E & J retooled its operations, talking to consumers, trying new, lightweight, plastic composites. Companies now market directly to consumers, through magazines, the Internet, and other venues. Compared to 30 years ago, today's wheelchair market has numerous options, with models to suit diverse needs—assuming the consumers can pay for their equipment.

Wheelchair Options

Wheelchair technologies span the gamut (see Figure 8.2). The old standard, chrome model with leatherette sling back and sling seat remains ubiquitous in institutions, as a means to ferry patients around. Since they are now comparatively inexpensive, these relatively heavy and uncomfortable wheelchairs are all some people can afford, even for home and community use. But for people with more money, numerous models exist, ranging from ultralightweight, three-wheeled chairs for marathoners to plastic chairs with bulbous wheels for rolling along sandy beaches to all-terrain, four-wheeled, power wheelchairs for traversing rugged surfaces to technologically sophisticated power wheelchairs controlled by pneumatic switches. Given this diversity, this brief description covers only wheelchair basics.

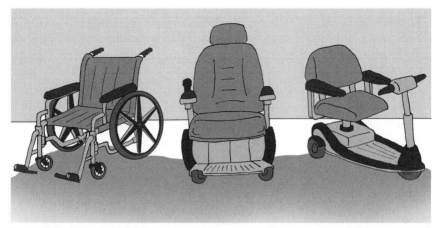

Figure 8.2. Wheeled Mobility Aids. This drawing illustrates three different types of wheelchairs (from left to right): manual wheelchair, which riders either self-propel or are pushed; power wheelchair, operated by batteries located at the rear under the seat; and a scooter, powered by batteries also under the seat. [Anil Shukla]

When selecting a wheelchair, the primary decision revolves around the degree of independence the user will have. Sophisticated technologies now allow even persons with severe physical debilities to operate power wheelchairs and move independently. Depending on individual circumstances, including cognitive functioning and judgment, the safest option may require someone to be accompanied and pushed in a wheelchair. Trading off independence for safety is complicated.

If people choose independence, deciding between manual and power wheelchairs depends primarily on having the physical strength and stamina to self-propel a manual chair. Most manual wheelchairs have push handles, so that other people can help tired users. But being pushed defeats the goal of being independent and in control. As wheelchair expert Gary Karp (1998) observed, people need to be honest with themselves about their levels of strength and energy, since self-propelling a manual wheelchair requires a lot of both.

Given concerns about fatigue, weakness, and heat sensitivity, most persons with MS choose power equipment for independence. Nonetheless, manual wheelchairs offer considerable advantages if someone has a willing push partner, including the following:

- Lighter weight (batteries are very heavy)
- Range limited only by the endurance of the wheelchair pusher, not by the charge capacity of a battery

- Lower purchase and maintenance price
- More discreet presence: less bulky and generates little noise (battery-powered equipment hums as it moves along)
- Easier to transport in cars, airplanes, trains, and buses (manual chairs fold flat or easily come apart into small pieces)
- Greater ability to surmount environmental barriers (persons who master the so-called wheelie can jump a curb or step; the wheelchair pusher can tip the wheelchair backward, lifting the user onto a curb).

Likely because of these advantages, many persons with MS acquire manual wheelchairs to use in selected settings and when someone is available to do the pushing. As we found in our survey of 703 persons with MS, manual wheelchairs were the most common mobility aid, owned by 53 percent of respondents compared with the 34 percent who owned canes (Iezzoni, Rao, and Kinkel, 2009). We also asked if people had not used specific mobility aids recently: 12 percent of manual wheelchair owners had not recently used this equipment, compared with 16 percent for canes.

For people without adequate strength or endurance to self-propel manual wheelchairs, battery-powered equipment—power wheelchairs and scooters—is liberating. Power wheelchairs offer the following advantages over manual chairs:

- Conserves energy and minimizes exhaustion
- Reduces the likelihood of needing assistance from others when traveling long distances, assuming the battery charge is sufficient
- Climbs uphill slopes that are not too steep
- Leaves one arm free to do other things
- Offers specialized technologies, such as powered tilt or reclining, which can lessen risk of pressure sores and improve comfort

After choosing between manual and power wheelchairs, many decisions remain, such as solid rubber versus pneumatic tires, fixed or swingaway footrests, seat depth and width, flat back versus lumbar back support, and type of cushions (including foam, gel, air flotation, or urethane honeycomb). Typically, wheelchairs and cushions are purchased separately, although they must function together as a team. Given these diverse options and the biomechanical ramifications of these decisions, working closely with knowledgeable rehabilitation professionals (see Chapter 7) to select the best equipment for meeting individual needs is important.

Manual Wheelchairs

Manual wheelchairs come in two major types: rigid frame and folding frame. Throughout history, the rigid, heavy frames of wooden wheelchairs severely impeded self-propulsion and travel. With recent advances in wheelchair technologies, engineers found that the flexible frames of collapsible wheelchairs consume energy. Pound for pound, collapsible wheelchairs take more effort to propel.

Engineers have designed rigid-frame wheelchairs, which have fewer moving parts without the folding frame device. Rigid-frame wheelchairs are very lightweight, strong, and energy efficient. They are streamlined and unobtrusive. But because they are extremely responsive, even minor movements of the rider's body can cause rigid-frame wheelchairs to change direction. Athletes find this sensitivity essential to their quick maneuverability, while others are unnerved by it. On uneven surfaces, rigid-frame wheelchairs give a bumpy ride and can become dangerous when one or more wheels lift off the ground. Rigid-frame wheelchairs do not fold neatly for easy storage, but they typically pop apart easily, permitting stowage in cars.

Despite their heavier weight, flexible-frame chairs offer some advantages over rigid-frame models. They fold easily for storage at home and in car trunks. They routinely have push handles just in case the user cannot self-propel (many rigid-frame chairs do not). They are safer on rough terrain because all four wheels are more likely to remain in contact with the ground. But given their greater weight, flexible-frame wheelchairs demand more energy to propel. After choosing between rigid- and flexible-frame wheelchairs, other decisions remain, including wheel size, placement and angle (camber) of wheels, width of handrims for self-propelling wheels, and wheel locks or hand brakes. These decisions must consider not only the height and strength of users but also their lifestyle and ways they plan to use the wheelchair.

Engineers continue to work on designing more functional manual wheelchairs. Power-assist pushrim-activated wheelchairs (PAPAW) are manual wheelchairs with battery-powered assistance for the pushrim: the circular frame affixed to the two large rear wheels that riders push to self-propel a manual wheelchair. In PAPAWs, a battery-powered device engages to help rotate or push the wheel, contributing energy to the rider's own efforts and boosting wheelchair propulsion forward. PAPAW wheels and power-assist devices can be fitted to most manual wheelchairs. PAPAW devices typically cost more than $5,000, and they add weight to manual wheelchairs. Nonetheless, this technology may be useful to persons with MS who want to use manual wheelchairs but need the energy boost for forward propulsion that the PAPAW device provides.

Power Wheelchairs and Scooters

Power wheelchairs and scooters use battery power to transport users. This makes powered equipment attractive to persons with MS, who typically lack the energy and strength for self-propelling manual wheelchairs long distances. Their different designs have important consequences, which potential users must consider in choosing between them (see Figure 8.2). Power wheelchairs roll on four (or more) wheels, with the battery power pack below the seat and flip-up footplates or swing-away footrest hangers. Users generally maneuver power wheelchairs using a short, vertical joystick positioned on the armrest. People unable to move their hands operate power wheelchairs equipped with sophisticated technologies that respond to puffs and sips of air blown through a straw-like device.

In contrast, the configuration of scooters—which is a type of wheelchair, given its function and purpose—resembles a cart (as Gerald Bernadine called his equipment) or vehicle, with the driver seated behind the controls. Scooters are built upon a platform, with a rotating captain's chair rising from the back, battery pack underneath the seat, and a steering column on the front. Scooter steering columns can carry a basket, horn, and/or headlight. Because of this configuration, scooters can carry packages and suitcases with little hindrance. When traveling, I tuck my suitcase on the platform underneath my legs and put smaller items in my basket. Users drive scooters by pulling or pressing levers on the handlebars, regulating speed with a dial (scooters generally travel at four or five miles per hour). Most scooters are three-wheeled, but because of their potential instability, four-wheeled versions are also available. Scooters are safe and appropriate only for people with good hand and arm strength and upper-body balance.

Both power wheelchairs and scooters come in two versions, either front- or rear-wheel drive: the drive wheels are positioned either in the front or back. (Some new power wheelchairs are mid-wheel drive.) Front-wheel drive equipment has a smaller turning radius, so people can rotate fully in tight spaces. Riders have the sensation of being pulled forward, so they must be alert to the chair's movements and surroundings. Surmounting low obstacles is easier, although the weight of power equipment generally precludes curb jumping. Rear-wheel models give a greater sense of control but need wider spaces for turning. Rear-wheel drive power wheelchairs can tip over when the front casters lift off the ground as heavy rear wheels accelerate.

Virtually all battery-powered wheelchairs and scooters sold today use nonspillable, rechargeable, lead-acid batteries. Batteries convert chemical energy into electrical energy through chemical reactions on the battery's plates or electrodes. In a rechargeable battery, an electric current reverses those chemical reactions.

An early rechargeable battery technology, such as that still used in cars, involves the lead-acid battery, which uses a liquid stored upright in an unsealed container, posing risks of spilling dangerous acid and emission of gases from the chemical reaction. In nonspillable batteries, instead of free liquid (sulfuric) acid, the battery acid is either in the form of a thick gel or (less commonly) is absorbed onto a glass fiber mat (so-called absorbed glass mat or AGM technology). The batteries are also sealed to eliminate any possibility of spilling corrosive chemicals, and a pressure relief valve prevents the buildup of internal gases.

Unlike car batteries, which are designed for a short-duration, high-power discharge, wheelchair and scooter batteries discharge their energy at a lower level but at approximately constant current, powering the device for sometimes many miles without requiring recharging. Many power wheelchairs and scooters now have internal recharging equipment. So at the end of the day, the user simply plugs the charger cord into a standard electrical outlet to fully charge the battery for the next day's use.

Keeping track of the battery charge is essential. Otherwise, problems can occur such as Gerald Bernadine had a few weeks after he got his scooter. "It went dead on me," Mr. Bernadine recalled. "I was zipping all over this place, and one day, it wouldn't go. I turned on the key, and I checked all the connections. Nothing seemed wrong. So my colleague helped me push it down to the car." That evening Mr. Bernadine finally read the instruction book. "I learned that I have to watch the battery level," he admitted ruefully. "Now every week I recharge my batteries."

Mr. Bernadine was fortunate that his power failure occurred at his office. Losing power can be terrifying, as happened to philosophy professor Toombs (1995, 15):

> I was crossing the plaza outside the university library when my scooter stopped dead in its tracks. I was surrounded by a sea of concrete embedded with decorative pebbles, marooned in the middle of a flat, completely open area with no trees, no lampposts, no benches anywhere within reach. I did not have my crutches. There was no one in sight. The nearest "object" was the building, but it was impossible to reach on my own two feet with nothing to support me. Nor could I easily crawl the distance, given the hard uneven surface of the pebbled cement. . . . The space of the plaza, which a moment before had been bright, sunny, inviting, now suddenly appeared ominous.

Toombs's misadventure occurred before people routinely carried cell phones, although Toombs did have a car phone in her van. In case of emergency, I always take my cell phone with me whenever I roll out on the streets. In my 21 years of using scooters, I have lost electrical power three times—most dramatically, one evening in the North Station stop of Boston's subway system. (That episode likely resulted from wires becoming disconnected after I rode over the bumpy terrain of uneven sidewalk and street pavement in Boston's West End.) Four subway employees helped get my dead scooter out of the station and onto a wheelchair-accessible taxi.

Despite these very rare lapses, battery-powered equipment allows persons with MS to "husband their energy," as one woman told me. "Sometimes I'm so tired I could drop," she said. "It's just not worth it to get exhausted. You have to take precautions, to conserve your energy. Using the scooter, that's husbanding my energy."

Fears of Dependence and Loss

As noted above, 85 percent of manual wheelchair users in our survey of 703 persons with MS were afraid of becoming dependent on their wheelchair: losing what little ability they had to walk. These fears focus on the potential for specific physical losses (leg strength and endurance), while champions of wheelchair use emphasize moving the whole person around independently and free from physical worries. People who fear dependence also underscore their psychic determination to endure and push on, to reject giving in.

Fears of dependence emanate from the dictum use-it-or-lose-it—that if you do not use your legs, you will lose whatever strength or ability your legs once had (Iezzoni, 2003). This position does have some veracity. Even elite athletes lose peak conditioning after several days without exercise. For many people with progressive chronic conditions such as MS, however, this belief isolates the legs from the whole person. It assumes that the primary objective is maximizing failing muscle function rather than considering the totality of a person's daily life. Those who look beyond use-it-or-lose-it focus on enhancing quality of life for the whole person.

People's frame of reference thus flips at some point, prompted by increasing physical limitations or frustration with existing limitations. They decide that the prospect of independence trumps fears of dependence, and they start using wheeled mobility aids. At that point many become less afraid—of falling or getting stuck when their legs fail. People who can still walk do walk whenever they can, using their wheelchair selectively. They do not see wheelchair use as an either or decision—they make choices daily.

For those able to make these choices, using a wheelchair must reconcile complicated and competing feelings, often reversing long-held images and substituting empowerment for loss. Sometimes other people, including family members, impose their own perspectives on these decisions. An experienced occupational therapist (OT) observed that some people with progressive chronic conditions, such as MS, contend that they are not yet ready for a wheelchair even when their debilities are severe. "It's so hard to accept the wheelchair," she said.

> I had a patient with MS. He was huge—a big guy. He'd been fine for years and years and then got worse. Another OT and I were trying to move him around his apartment, and we were holding him up with all our weight. We were praying to God—you could see both of us looking up to the sky. If this guy went down, the police were getting called because there was no way we were lifting this guy off the floor. We finally got him to get a power wheelchair.

Now the man can get around on his own.

PAYING FOR MOBILITY AIDS

Costs of mobility aids rise with increasing technological complexity. Although persons can purchase simple canes for $20 or less at the local drugstore, rolling walkers with handlebar brakes and seats can cost $150 to $250. A good quality manual wheelchair with adequate cushioning and back supports can cost $1,500 to $2,000, scooters can run $2,000 to $5,000, and power wheelchairs start at $5,000. Sophisticated power wheelchairs, with seats that raise and tilt and other computer-operated features, can cost up to $30,000. Not surprisingly, therefore, many persons turn to health insurance for financial assistance in acquiring mobility aids.

Medicare—the federal health insurance program for elderly and disabled persons—is the dominant force in the mobility aid health insurance marketplace. Medicare policies drive both the actions of private health insurers and the nature and, increasingly, the products offered by mobility aid manufacturers. This brief review of health insurance coverage policies for mobility aids therefore focuses on Medicare.

Health Insurance Basics

Health insurance never covers all items or services. Instead, the purchaser of the health insurance—such as the federal government for Medicare—decides which items and services the insurance will cover. Those decisions circumscribe the so-called benefit package. The broader the benefit package, the more costly the health insurance. Therefore, the first question to ask is: does the health insurance benefit package cover mobility aids?

Even if an item or service is part of the health insurance benefit package, insurers often set rules to determine who qualifies for coverage of specific items or services within this benefit package. For example, if health insurance covers mobility aids, the insurer may place restrictions on which individuals qualify for the coverage (so-called individual coverage decisions). So the second question to ask is, does this particular individual qualify for the specific type of mobility aid that is considered a covered item or service?

Medicare is the federal health insurance program for persons who are age 65 and older (almost all elderly qualify, with a few narrow exceptions), persons of all ages with end-stage renal disease requiring dialysis or kidney transplant, and former workers who have qualified for Social Security Disability Insurance (SSDI) and have met other criteria (such as a 24-month wait following first SSDI cash payments; see Chapter 9). Many persons with MS eventually acquire Medicare, either by aging into the system or through SSDI.

Medicare Coverage of Mobility Aids

Federal statutes set the broad boundaries of Medicare's benefit package. By federal laws, Medicare covers only those items and services deemed "medically necessary," defined as "reasonable and necessary for the diagnosis or treatment of illness or injury or to improve the functioning of a malformed body member" (42 C.F.R. Sec. 402.3). Federal statutes also exclude items deemed to be primarily for personal comfort or convenience. For so-called durable medical equipment (DME), which includes mobility aids, Medicare adds one further stipulation: the program pays for the rental or purchase of this equipment only "if the equipment is used in the patient's home or in an institution that is used as a home" (42 C.F.R. Sec. 410.38(a)). Assisting mobility *outside* the home is considered a convenience and not medically necessary.

Medicare has additional rules about qualifying for a power wheelchair or scooter, which Medicare calls a power-operated vehicle or POV. In addition to needing to use the equipment inside the home to perform routine daily activities (such as toileting, bathing, and dressing), the patient must demonstrate the physical, cognitive, and visual/perceptual skills needed to safely operate the POV within the home environment. Specifically, a physician must certify to Medicare that the person can operate the equipment safely. In addition, the home environment must be accessible to the power wheelchair or scooter, as documented by a home visit by the DME supplier or a rehabilitation therapist.

Implications of Medicare Coverage Policies for Persons with MS

The requirement of needing wheeled mobility aids to perform daily activities—toileting, feeding, dressing, grooming, and bathing—and stipulation of in-home use poses problems for many Medicare beneficiaries with MS who seek coverage for mobility aids. Certainly, a small fraction of persons with MS are permanently unable to ambulate at all and require wheeled mobility aids (powered or not) to move any distance. However, most persons with MS who have impaired mobility have sufficient ability, using ambulation aids or by wall walking or furniture surfing, to manage within their homes. Furthermore, a person's ability to perform these daily activities can change from month to month or vary depending on time of day, such as early morning versus late afternoon. Thus, depending on the severity of impairment, establishing a person's mobility status in the home may not be clear-cut.

To ensure their patients get needed equipment, neurologists must therefore evaluate a person's needs based on their worst days, such as a steamy hot summer day when the person is tired from previous activity. Neurologists therefore ask patients, "On your worst days, can you safely make it to your front door in a timely fashion?" The answer to this question can assist in determining the person's qualification for powered mobility aids under Medicare. In asking such practical questions, the size of a person's home (the distances they must travel) may determine need.

The same person with identical impairments may give two entirely different but equally honest answers depending on where he or she lives. For example, in a small one bedroom apartment with narrow hallways, the person gets around fine. The person can use an external support for almost any step—touching the walls, holding onto the backs of chairs, grabbing the doorframe, moving from bedroom to bathroom to kitchen—without falling. In contrast, the same person in a large home, with wide interior spaces, may have trouble getting to the front door safely and efficiently on a bad day. Without anything to hold on to, the person may fall or be too fatigued or imbalanced to get to the door on his or her legs. If the home is accessible (has wide doorways, ample maneuvering room, ramps; see Chapter 9), the person in the large home may qualify for a scooter or a power wheelchair designed for use inside the home.

For those who need a powered mobility aid in their home, Medicare policies do not prohibit outdoor use of the equipment. Challenges come when the features, functions, and durability of the equipment do not meet outdoor mobility demands. A small scooter, with limited battery capacity, may be insufficient to reliably go the distances required to do errands outside the home. Medicare's benefit package does not cover equipment designed for outdoor, long-distance use.

Implications of Medicare Policies for Mobility Aid Products

Although Medicare's various policy activities might appear distant from manufacturing lines and bioengineering research laboratories, they have significant effects on inventors and producers of mobility aids. Because Medicare is the dominant purchaser of DME, Medicare policy changes and fee schedules affect mobility aid manufacturers throughout the entire public and private marketplace. A strong belief has arisen in the field that innovation and discovery, especially involving new designs for powered equipment and associated technologies (e.g., batteries), have suffered from Medicare's reimbursement policies and focus on equipment for use only in homes.

Within the last several years, limitations on Medicare reimbursement levels for mobility aids have resulted in disincentives for innovation and development of new products by wheelchair manufacturers. In contrast, these limits have strengthened incentives to manufacture products that meet the minimal standards sufficient for in-home use. Products designed for in-home use only are not as durable or reliable as products designed for community mobility needs. The downstream effects of Medicare policy decisions on the wheelchair industry are evident when traveling outside the United States, especially to western European and certain Asian countries. The range of mobility aid product options and innovation available to western European and some Asian consumers greatly outstrips the products sold in the United States. Often mobility aids available through an American-based, multinational company are far more extensive in Europe or Asia than in the United States. When asked why various products are not available to American consumers, the manufacturer's answer is simple: Medicare's payment levels are too low.

An example of how Medicare payment policy undercut a new technology coming into the market is the iBOT® power wheelchair, which as of January 2009 was no longer being sold by its manufacturer, Independence Technology L.L.C. Dean Kamen (who also invented the Segway Personal Transporter) invented iBOT in a partnership between DEKA Research & Development Corporation and Johnson & Johnson Company. iBOT has two sets of powered wheels that rotate around each other on either side of the chair, allowing the equipment to climb stairs. Various sensors and gyroscopes, operated by sophisticated software, stabilize the wheelchair, allowing users to mount curbs, traverse uneven ground, and rise to standing height. iBOT cost just over $26,000.

As a new technology, iBOT received approval from the U.S. Food and Drug Administration, qualifying as a Class 2 medical device. However, for payment purposes, Medicare assigned iBOT to the Group 3 payment category, which covers standard function power wheelchairs. Medicare viewed all other functions of iBOT, such as the ability to climb stairs and rise to standing height, as convenience items, which are not covered under Medicare's statutes (see above). Group 3 reimbursement level fell far below the costs of producing iBOT, making it financially impossible to provide iBOT to Medicare beneficiaries. The price tag also put iBOT beyond the resources of the average wheelchair user—few could afford to pay $26,000 themselves. Without Medicare coverage and private insurance support, the manufacturer stopped making iBOTs.

Persons with MS who can get around their homes without powered mobility aids are likely to be disappointed when suppliers or therapists indicate that Medicare will not pay for the scooter or power wheelchair they might want for use outside the home. However, that is the reality of today's Medicare coverage policies. Those individuals can still purchase this equipment themselves. But for persons on fixed incomes, such as monthly disability payments, powered mobility aids costing potentially several thousand dollars may be beyond their reach. Medicaid, the joint federal and state health insurance program for persons who are poor and disabled (among others), has somewhat more generous wheelchair allowances than Medicare (although specific policies vary from state to state). But Medicaid also would not pay for the stair-climbing iBOT.

9

Accommodating Disability and Disability Civil Rights

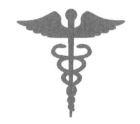

J oe Alto had operated a backhoe on construction sites before being diagnosed with MS in his mid-twenties (Iezzoni and O'Day, 2006). He had to leave his job because he no longer had the physical stamina for the work. With only a high school education and no specialized job skills, he had few other career options. Mr. Alto was able to scrape by financially with monthly checks from a federal income support program for people with disabilities. For the first several years, he had relapsing-remitting MS and got around using forearm crutches to stabilize his gait. By his late twenties, Mr. Alto's MS had progressed to the point where he could barely walk.

But Mr. Alto didn't get a wheelchair. He lived in an apartment building with stairs going to the front door and no accessible entrance (entryway that wheelchair users could roll through, free from physical barriers). The apartment building also had no elevator—only stairs—and Joe lived on the fourth floor. Even if he'd had a wheelchair, Joe would have been unable to get into or out of his apartment using it. Because of this, Joe said, "I was stuck in my house for ten years."

Mr. Alto felt that things could have been worse. He was hospitalized several times for MS flares, and he was terrified that nurses and doctors would find out about his inaccessible housing. "If you're disabled and can't go up and down the stairs, and you live in an apartment without an elevator," said Joe, "the hospital will send you to a nursing home. They're not supposed to send you home." Being forced into a nursing home was his greatest fear. After considerable effort, Joe finally found an accessible (barrier-free) apartment and got his power wheelchair.

Despite this eventual resolution, Joe Alto's 10-year forced isolation in an inaccessible home took a heavy toll. It likely led to profound depression, a secondary disability (a disability on top of his walking impairment) that was possibly preventable if only he'd had an accessible apartment and appropriate mobility aid. "If you tell a person they can't do nothing, that's like telling them to go home and die," Joe observed. "If you lose hope, you don't want to live no more."

Luckily, Mr. Alto's wheelchair and new accessible home restored his optimism and sense of mission. Joe now aims to educate everyone he possibly can about building accessible environments—not just homes but also public and private buildings, transportation systems (buses and subways), and other spaces people use in everyday life. He recently chalked up a major victory with his dentist: "I couldn't get into his office with my wheelchair, so I talked to him. And he built a ramp!" According to Mr. Alto, if people speak up, accessibility will improve.

* * * * *

As noted throughout this book, MS typically strikes people early in their lives, just as they are starting families, entering the labor force, building careers, and looking forward to their futures. Because MS is currently incurable, many persons can anticipate living for decades with a condition that frequently becomes disabling as the years pass by. But as Joe Alto said, "If you lose hope, you don't want to live no more."

Everybody with MS finds his or her own way to live with the disease. The social and physical environments within which people live determine, to a large extent, how rich and varied those lives will be. The resiliency of individuals—their innate, inborn ability to bounce back and rise above psychic trauma and physical hardship—obviously plays a huge role. But if someone is stuck in an inaccessible apartment for 10 years, as was Joe Alto, even the most resilient and resourceful persons would likely suffer the depression that afflicted Joe. The transformation of his environment made all the difference. Joe Alto's wheelchair and accessible apartment restored his sense of purpose in the world. He became a man with a mission.

This final chapter looks at various social and physical environmental factors that affect the lives of all persons with disabilities, not only individuals with MS. Because MS often affects persons so early in life, however, these environmental attributes play an especially huge role for people with MS. For each individual, the relative importance of one social or physical environmental factor versus another will vary based on their personal circumstances. But all these factors affect virtually everyone with MS to some degree at some point in their lives. The chapter ends by returning to my own experiences with MS.

THE ONION

One can imagine that the various critical social and physical environmental factors are like the layers of an onion, building outward from a core. The individual with MS resides at that central core. Wrapping most closely around the individual is the home and close family. Just outside that layer are friends and other relatives. Beyond that layer are the workplace and colleagues, for those still able to work. Then comes the local community: churches and other houses of worship, stores, schools, transportation systems, post offices, banks, restaurants, beauty salons, movie theaters, parks and recreational facilities, hospitals and doctor's offices, and other places people go to run errands, share spiritual and recreational time with family and friends, and do the other activities essential to daily life.

Beyond the local community are governmental laws and policies, at the state and national levels, that mandate basic income support and civil rights (including employment rights) for persons with disabilities. These laws and policies also determine important aspects of the physical environment, such as accessibility of transportation systems, city sidewalks, public and private buildings, and businesses. Although these laws and policies might seem very distant from the individual at the onion's core, they can affect daily life in specific and critical ways. Joe Alto, for instance, gets monthly payments from a federal disability insurance plan (Supplemental Security Income or SSI) that provides income support to persons who are poor and disabled and can no longer work. He uses this money to buy food, pay his rent, and meet other necessary expenses. By qualifying for SSI, Mr. Alto also gets Medicaid, a joint federal and state health insurance program for poor and disabled persons, among others. In addition, Mr. Alto rides the subway to visit his neurologist. The subway is now required by law to be accessible to persons with disabilities. Before this law (and a lawsuit filed by people with disabilities to enforce the law), the subway system had no elevators or trains accessible to wheelchair users.

Finally, the outermost layer of the onion is societal attitudes. Historically, society stigmatized persons with disabilities, largely hiding them away and discriminating against them in numerous ways. Societal attitudes are particularly felt by persons who use wheelchairs—that most visible sign of disability—as they go out into the community, deal with strangers (such as store clerks and restaurant wait staff), and encounter passersby on the streets. Being made fun of, disregarded, or treated disrespectfully because of using a wheelchair is degrading and discouraging. Although many of us are exhorted from an early age to nurture our own sense of self-worth and value, this is hard to do and maintain in the face of constantly disparaging societal attitudes.

The effects of all these various layers of the environmental onion are mitigated by two major contextual factors: education and income. Persons who are well educated and have high incomes can often find ways to transcend or rise above impediments posed at different junctures of the social and physical environments. Highly educated individuals have more employment options, especially work that does not require exhausting manual labor. Persons with substantial financial resources can afford to renovate their homes to improve physical accessibility or move to new, more accommodating housing. Interestingly, persons with MS tend to have relatively high education attainment, as suggested by findings from the Sonya Slifka study introduced in Chapter 2 (see Table 9.1). Compared with the general U.S. population, however, their incomes are somewhat lower, possibly because far fewer persons with MS are employed. Persons with MS are much more likely to be married than persons in the general population.

The onion metaphor presented here parallels closely the so-called determinants of health model, which is driving the federal Healthy People 2020 public health initiative: efforts to improve the health and well-being of Americans during the next decade (www.healthypeople.gov/HP2020). The determinants of health approach believes that many factors affect people's health, including their genetic traits and personal attributes, such as age, sex, race, and disease. In addition—and importantly—social and physical environmental factors that cut across individuals play critical roles. Examples of environmental hazards that determine population health include widespread and endemic poverty, causing general stress and hopelessness; dilapidated and decaying housing; limited availability of fresh fruits and vegetables in local stores, resulting in unhealthy diets; poor air and water quality; neighborhoods rife with crime where people are afraid to walk outdoors and exercise, contributing to persons becoming obese or overweight; and the absence of green spaces and parks for recreation and leisure activities.

The discussion below examines several layers of the onion, starting with the outermost skin: societal attitudes. The chapter then considers civil rights laws, income support policies, and public transportation for persons with disabilities. Going deeper, the chapter then addresses employment and accommodations that might assist persons with MS. The onion review concludes by delving into that most intimate layer—the home and family relationships.

Table 9.1
Education, Income, Employment, and Marital Status of Persons with MS Compared with the General Population in the United States

Characteristic	Persons with MS	General U.S. Population
Education		
Less than high school	4%	7%
High school graduate	23	41
1–3 years of college	33	27
College graduate	24	16
Postgraduate education	16	9
Family income (dollars per year)		
<$10,000	7	5
$10,000–$24,999	10	15
$25,000–$49,999	38	29
≥$50,000	45	51
Employment		
In the labor force	44	66
Not in the labor force	56	34
Marital status		
Married	67	57
Divorced or separated	18	11
Never married	10	30
Widowed	5	2

Adapted from Minden et al., 2006.

SOCIETAL ATTITUDES

Today, a diverse and extensive array of disability-related activities is occurring. Centers for Independent Living (CILs), run by people with disabilities in numerous locations around the country, bolster consumer empowerment and community advocacy; state and local governments sponsor offices to address issues relating to disability; disability rights centers offer legal counsel and advocacy; hundreds of Internet sites provide disability-related services, advice, information, and support; numerous companies market products, ranging from customized wheelchairs to cars with hand controls to accessible vacations; wheelchair users roll through television shows, commercials, and movies; dance troupes and other cultural organizations feature artists using wheelchairs; elite athletes compete in Paralympic Games and numerous other sporting events; and a vibrant community of disability studies scholars carefully observes and chronicles societal attitudes. People with disabilities can find themselves not only included but celebrated.

Despite this, many attitudes toward people with disabilities remain a complex tangle of fears, discomforts, sorrows, and uncertainties. Much of society still holds people with disabilities individually responsible for problems in conducting daily activities (such as difficulties with employment, transportation, and housing), rather than organizing the world to accommodate disability. Sometimes these discomforts spill out into the open, as strangers tell us their perceptions. Early one morning at Boston's Logan Airport, I was waiting in my scooter in the security screening line, and a man walked up to me. He was a wheelchair pusher whom I'd spoken to before. Short and dapper, he had told me of his pride that his hair was only lightly touched by grey despite his 65 years. "Can you tell me," he asked that morning, "what is wrong with you?" He seemed genuinely concerned—although pointedly curious—and in most such situations these days, I try to see educational opportunities.

"I have MS. Multiple sclerosis." He still looked perplexed. "A disease of the nerves."

He reached to a cord around his neck and fished out a cross. "Jesus, Mary, and Joseph," he said, kissing the cross. "Can it be cured?"

"No," I said.

"I'm Italian," he said, "I'll pray for you." He walked away, shaking his head.

Historical Perspective

Society's views of disabilities are deep-rooted, often dark, and complicated. Leviticus, in the Old Testament of the Bible, catalogued the "blemishes" that precluded persons from joining religious ceremonies. This list included "a man blind or lame, or one who has a mutilated face or a limb too long, or a man who has an injured foot or an injured hand, or a hunchback, or a dwarf . . . ."

As societies developed, they depended on people to work to support themselves and their families, as well as to give something back to their communities. Societies acknowledged that not everyone is able to work to meet their needs.

In these instances, communities must help out. Human nature, however, posed a problem. Some people were lazy and avoided work by exaggerating or fabricating physical problems. Even hundreds of years ago, societies decided they needed to figure out ways to separate out the meritorious person with true disabilities from people who were faking impairments (Stone, 1984).

Fourteenth-century English laws held that the so-called honest beggar came involuntarily to his plight, forced by circumstances beyond his control. In England, from the sixteenth through nineteenth centuries, reports circulated of vagrants self-mutilating and feigning impairments. In France, some beggars allegedly learned medicine to make their duplicitous ailments appear more realistic. By late-nineteenth-century England, the focus shifted to vocational training for deserving disabled people, nonetheless called "the defectives." Simultaneously, social Darwinism and the eugenics movement emerged, questioning whether society should even include disabled members. The belief that most human characteristics are inherited, including impairments, became the rationale for Adolf Hitler's so-called euthanasia program, which killed over 200,000 Germans with disabilities starting in 1939.

In seventeenth-century America, the physical challenges of exploring and settling a rough and rugged country resulted in early colonists prizing physical stamina. Initial settlers fought against the immigration of persons who might need community support. Potentially dependent people with physical or mental impairments could be deported, sent back to their home countries. By the time of the Revolutionary War, these views had eased somewhat. Despite this, in early America, Protestantism led to moralistic views of misfortune, with clerics and laity alike believing that sin predisposed persons to illness (Starr, 1982). Women were expected to care for sickness, keeping it hidden in the home. Exceptions to these attitudes involved injured military personnel. In 1798, the federal government established marine hospitals for sick and disabled sailors. Roughly 60,000 amputations were performed during the Civil War, about 40 percent involving lower extremities (Figg and Farrell-Beck, 1993). In 1862, Congress passed the first of several laws to assist disabled veterans, including federal grants of $75 to Union soldiers to purchase an artificial leg. Southern states bore these expenses for Confederate veterans.

By mid-twentieth-century America, beliefs had shifted from moralistic to biological explanations for disability, but persons with disabilities still remained hidden in homes, rarely emerging into public view. Into this societal environment came Franklin Delano Roosevelt, who contracted polio at age 39 (see Chapter 8). In August 1921 at his Campobello resort after visiting a boy scout camp, Roosevelt experienced the earliest sign of impending polio, an evening chill. By the next day, he was unable to walk, and Roosevelt never took another true step. He also never complained or even talked about his impairment to friends or family, including his wife Eleanor. For seven years after his illness, he struggled, without success, to walk the length of his driveway at Hyde Park, New York.

How much Roosevelt deceived himself remains unclear, but he knew he must deceive Americans to achieve his political ambitions. People would reject a non-walking leader. Roosevelt therefore created a fiction (Gallagher, 1994). After arduous practice, Roosevelt appeared to walk when he actually threw his legs sequentially forward from the hips while being carried forward by his bent elbow (on one side) and weight-bearing cane (on the other side).

At the time, Roosevelt's denial of his disability served his nation well. Before polio, Roosevelt had appeared cocky and arrogant; after polio, he understood pain and connected with people. The public accepted the fiction that Roosevelt had overcome polio and was now just a little lame. Even the White House photography corps hid Roosevelt's wheelchair use. When uncooperative photographers tried sneaking a shot, other photographers would seemingly accidentally knock their cameras or block their views. Secret Service agents seized film from people violating the unspoken code by photographing the president. From the unseen wheelchair and almost without respite, Roosevelt led the nation through its darkest days in the twentieth century.

Roosevelt's legacy relating to disability is complicated. Eleanor Roosevelt reportedly conceded that her husband never admitted he could not walk (Gallagher, 1998, 208). Yet almost from the moment the original Social Security Act passed in 1935, Roosevelt contemplated expanding the program and adding medical and disability benefits. During World War II, disabled persons (including women) worked in record numbers because of wartime demands, although they lost these positions when the war ended. With hindsight bolstered by pop psychology, Roosevelt's denial of his disability was undoubtedly deep. Especially among the World War II generation, however, Roosevelt's attitudes resonated, perhaps exemplifying the vaunted national persona—tough, independent, not complaining, and getting the job done. But with Roosevelt's silence, a moment was lost to teach the nation about how persons with disabilities could make essential and invaluable contributions to society.

Changing Attitudes

In his history of the disability rights movement in the United States, journalist Joseph Shapiro (1994) gives substantial credit to efforts to reintegrate injured World War II veterans into society. With Roosevelt's support and the

G.I. Bill—an educational grant program for returning World War II veterans, nicknamed G.I.s—even disabled veterans sought training at colleges, universities, and vocational programs. Educational institutions nationwide made themselves accessible to welcome returning military personnel, including persons with disabilities.

An equally potent force was parents advocating for their children with disabilities. Groups such as the United Cerebral Palsy Association and Muscular Dystrophy Association, founded by parents in 1948 and 1950, respectively, pushed for better education and social supports for their children, who until then had often been placed in institutions. Education policy for children became a critical beachhead for disability rights.

Starting in the 1960s, the growing disability rights movement emphasized independent living in communities, shifting away from segregation within institutions or homes toward inclusion—making entire communities and the necessities of daily life accessible to persons with disabilities. The late Edward V. Roberts, sometimes called the father of the independent living movement, instigated this change as a student at the University of California–Berkeley in the early 1960s. Roberts was paralyzed from polio at age 14 and required a mechanical ventilator to breathe. He sued to gain admission to this prestigious university, which rejected his application. Once there, he formed a political action group called the Rolling Quads, which aspired to make Berkeley barrier-free. (The word quad is a play on quadriplegic, which means paralysis in all four limbs.) Their ultimate goal was to maximize independence and self-reliance of persons with disabilities who previously lived in isolation and dependence. Roberts later recalled,

> We secured the first curb cut in the country; it was at the corner of Bancroft and Telegraph Avenue. When we first talked to legislators about the issue, they told us, "Curb cuts, why do you need curb cuts? We never see people with disabilities out on the street. Who is going to use them?" They didn't understand that their reasoning was circular. When curb cuts were put in, they discovered that access for disabled people benefits many others as well. For instance, people pushing strollers use curb cuts, as do people on bikes and elderly people who can't lift their legs so high. So many people benefit from this accommodation. This is what the concept of universal design is all about. (Fleischer and Zames, 2001, 40)

Design, or sometimes redesign to eliminate barriers and ensure access, became central to ensuring civil rights for persons with disabilities. The universal design principles espoused by Roberts urged designs that would work for everyone—

persons with all sorts of abilities and disabilities. As he noted, curb cuts in sidewalks help not only wheelchair users but also a range of other people, including cyclists and parents pushing children in strollers. Disability rights advocates viewed inaccessible buildings, sidewalks, transportation systems, and other structures as a form of segregation, representing discrimination.

Civil rights legislation from the 1960s barring discrimination based on race, ethnicity, and gender sought to ignore these characteristics, striving to judge people based on individual merit without recognizing the trait that stigmatized them (the color of their skin or their gender). But disability rights advocates recognized that ignoring disability would not achieve their goal. Instead, disability must first be acknowledged, then the path to civil rights cleared by tearing down barriers.

CIVIL RIGHTS LAWS FOR PERSONS WITH DISABILITIES

The hard-won achievements of racial and ethnic minorities and women in the mid-1960s offered little to persons with disabilities. The Civil Rights Act of 1964, signed by President Lyndon B. Johnson, stated that all persons regardless of "race, color, religion, or national origin" are entitled to "full and equal enjoyment of the goods, services, privileges, advantages, and accommodations of any place of public accommodation." It did not refer to people with disabilities.

History of the Disability Civil Rights Movement

The political climate of the late 1960s and early 1970s shifted against broadening rights, with President Richard M. Nixon pledging to halt civil rights expansions and dismantle President Johnson's War on Poverty. In 1972, Minnesota Senator Hubert H. Humphrey tried unsuccessfully to add disability as a protected class to the Civil Rights Act. During this period of backlash against civil rights expansions, the fight for disability rights became largely an underground movement. The earliest major victory was Section 504 of the Rehabilitation Act of 1973, which was viewed as a stealth measure snuck into legislation.

> Section 504 of the Rehabilitation Act of 1973 was no more than a legislative afterthought . . . At the very end of the bill were tacked on four unnoticed provisions—the most important of which was Section 504—that made it illegal for any federal agency, public university, defense or other federal contractor, or any other institution or activity that received federal funding to discriminate against anyone "solely by reason of . . . handicap."
>
> . . . Congressional aides could not even remember who had suggested adding the civil rights protection. But the wording clearly was copied

straight out of the Civil Rights Act of 1964, which ruled out discrimination in federal programs on the basis of race, color, or national origin. There had been no hearings and no debate about Section 504, Members of Congress were either unaware of it or considered it "little more than a platitude" for a sympathetic group . . . . (Shapiro, 1994, 65)

Passage of Section 504 catalyzed a chain of events leading ultimately to the disability rights movement in the United States finding its voice. For four years, successive administrations (first under President Gerald Ford and then under President Jimmy Carter) resisted issuing regulations to implement Section 504, fearing its scope and potential costs. In April 1977, frustrated disability rights activists, led by wheelchair users, took over federal offices in San Francisco and held them for 25 days. When one administration official suggested setting up "separate but equal" facilities for disabled people, the proposal, with its unfortunate phraseology redolent of Jim Crow (discrimination against African Americans in the Deep South), backfired. The civil disobedience tactics surprised the nation but won this particular battle for disability rights advocates.

The Americans with Disabilities Act (ADA) was not enacted until many other battles were fought. Perhaps the biggest hurdle was fears about its costs, potential litigation, and burden on business. Unlike other civil rights legislation, the ADA requires that businesses and government do more than just stop discriminatory actions (Young, 1997). They must also take active steps to offer equal opportunity to persons with disabilities, as commensurate with their financial resources.

As Ronald Reagan's vice president, George H. W. Bush became an ADA supporter only after being pitched conservative arguments by a prominent Republican attorney, Evan J. Kemp, Jr., who used a power wheelchair and had himself been denied dozens of jobs. Kemp convinced Bush that persons with disabilities wanted independence and to get off welfare and into paying jobs. Some observers believe that disability rights leaders reached an unspoken agreement with conservative members of Congress. The agreement gave the civil rights protections with the expectation that newly empowered persons with disabilities would no longer need welfare assistance.

Eventually, President George H. W. Bush, whose family had been tragically touched by illness (his young daughter had died of cancer), emerged as a critical proponent of the legislation. But countless others made their strong voices heard. Admittedly, the law's passage evoked fractious debates, vocal protests, and uneasy and shifting alliances. Disability rights advocates represented wide-ranging constituencies, including persons who are deaf or blind and those with learning disabilities or physical impairments. This diversity complicated efforts to find common ground. Ultimately, though, the power of the disability rights movement came from the fact that most people—presidents, senators, and representatives, Democrats and Republicans, administration officials, and citizens—either have a disability or know someone with a disability. The cause seemed universal.

At the ADA's signing ceremony on July 26, 1990, the rhetoric soared. In his invocation (unusual at a bill signing), the Reverend Harold H. Wilke, who was born without arms, prayed, "From ancient times to today we celebrate the breaking of the chains holding your people in bondage." (After signing the bill, President Bush passed the signing pen to Reverend Wilke, who took it using his feet.) President Bush recalled the Fourth of July celebration three weeks previously, then called the signing day another Independence Day, as "every man, woman and child with a disability can now pass through once-closed doors into a bright new era of equality, independence and freedom" (Young, 1997, 231).

Provisions of the ADA

Once he got his power wheelchair and became a man with a mission—improving physical accessibility in his community—Joe Alto knew he needed to learn about the law. "If you're not knowledgeable about the ADA, about reasonable accommodations, they'll walk all over you," Mr. Alto asserted. He went to a CIL in town that focused on supporting communities of color (Mr. Alto is African American). During multiple CIL visits, his purpose was "to study the ADA, to learn about the law. That way, if I tell people I want reasonable accommodations, they'll think I know what I'm talking about."

According to its opening statement, the goal of the Americans with Disabilities Act (P.L. 101-336) is "to establish a clear and comprehensive prohibition of discrimination on the basis of disability." Title I of the ADA requires the Equal Employment Opportunity Commission, established by the Civil Rights Act of 1964, to ensure that employers do not discriminate because of disability against otherwise qualified individuals "in regard to job application procedures, the hiring, advancement, or discharge of employees, employee compensation, job training, and other terms, conditions, and privileges of employment" (Sec. 102(a)). Discrimination includes "not making reasonable accommodations to the known physical or mental impairment" (Sec. 102(b)(5)(A)). Title II prohibits discrimination or denial of services provided by public entities, while Title III prohibits discrimination involving public accommodations and services operated by private entities.

The ADA used an expansive definition of disability (see Table 9.2). Unlike the approach of Title VII of the Civil Rights Act of 1964, the ADA forbids discrimination against "an individual with a disability," rather than against anyone (the entire group of people) with a disability. This means that individual claimants must first prove that they are, in fact, disabled before courts will hear their cases (Illingworth and Parmet, 2000). Only after they have proven to the court that they are disabled can claimants raise their accusation of discrimination. As shown in Table 9.2, regulations written to implement the ADA included MS among conditions that would constitute impairments under the law.

In several high-visibility and controversial ADA cases, however, the U.S. Supreme Court interpreted the law's broad definition of what constitutes

Table 9.2
Defining Disability in the Text and Regulations of the Americans with Disabilities Act

---

ADA Congressional Findings
Sec. 2(7) "...Individuals with disabilities are a discrete and insular minority who have been faced with restrictions and limitations, subjected to a history of purposeful unequal treatment, and relegated to a position of political powerlessness in our society, based on characteristics that are beyond the control of such individuals and resulting from stereotypic assumptions not truly indicative of the individual ability of such individuals to participate in, and contribute to, society; ... "

ADA Definitions
Sec. 3(2) "The term 'disability' means, with respect to an individual—(A) a physical or mental impairment that substantially limits one or more of the major life activities of such individual; (B) a record of such an impairment; or (C) being regarded as having such an impairment."
Sec. 101(8) "The term 'qualified individual with a disability' means an individual with a disability who, with or without reasonable accommodation, can perform the essential functions of the employment position ... "

Definitions in ADA Regulations: 28 CFR Part 36, Sec. 36.104
"It is not possible to include a list of all the specific conditions ... that would constitute physical or mental impairments ... However, [examples include]: Orthopedic, visual, speech and hearing impairments; cerebral palsy; epilepsy, muscular dystrophy, multiple sclerosis, cancer, heart disease, diabetes, mental retardation, emotional illness, specific learning disabilities, HIV [human immunodeficiency virus] disease (symptomatic or asymptomatic), tuberculosis, drug addiction, and alcoholism."
"Major life activities include such things as caring for one's self, performing manual tasks, walking, seeing, hearing, speaking, breathing, learning, and working."
To be substantially limited, an individual's important life activities must be "restricted as to the conditions, manner, or duration under which they can be performed in comparison to most people."

---

disability very narrowly. In *Toyota Motor Manufacturing Inc. v. Williams*, decided by a unanimous vote on January 8, 2002, the Supreme Court ruled against Ella Williams, who claimed that her carpal tunnel syndrome prevented her from performing her job at a Toyota manufacturing plant. The justices decided that Ms. Williams was not disabled because she could still perform routine tasks at home, such as brushing her teeth and gardening. In other words, the justices asserted, her condition did not limit major life activities. Despite her carpal tunnel syndrome, Ms. Williams was therefore not qualified to bring a lawsuit under the ADA. This ruling seemed to place employment-related activities outside the bounds of major life activities.

This and other Supreme Court decisions about disability qualifications filtered down to courts nationwide. Congress heard from numerous people with MS, diabetes, cancer, epilepsy, and other health problems that courts were denying them recognition as persons with disabilities. They were especially likely to be denied recognition as disabled if they took medications that controlled their conditions. This denial meant that these people could not get their day in court. Upset about these narrow interpretations of who qualifies as disabled under the ADA, Congress enacted new legislation—the Americans with Disabilities Act Amendments Act (ADAAA)—which President George W. Bush signed on September 25, 2008. The ADAAA, which won broad bipartisan approval (it passed by voice vote in the House and unanimous consent in the Senate) explicitly broadens the definition of who is qualified and eligible to bring lawsuits under the ADA. The ADAAA overrules the Supreme Court's strict limits on defining disability for ADA purposes.

The notion of making so-called reasonable accommodations for persons with disabilities had first arisen during litigation under Section 504 of the Rehabilitation Act of 1973, which first introduced broad federal disability rights (see above). The reasonable accommodation concept delineates the actions required to provide access to persons with disabilities that would not generate prohibitive expense or extraordinary effort. Under Section 504 lawsuits, courts at all levels had found that disabilities and potential accommodations are too diverse to develop a single standard for what is reasonable across all cases and all settings. Individual solutions are therefore necessary. The ADA adopted this practical framework.

By encompassing both private and public sectors, the ADA generated much more heated and complicated responses than did Section 504, which focused specifically on federal government programs and facilities. Anti-ADA sentiments arose almost immediately. Unlike other civil rights legislation, the ADA requires businesses to make reasonable accommodations for persons with disabilities. Businesses assumed this would be very expensive.

Some accommodations cost nothing, as when the U.S. Supreme Court on May 29, 2001, ruled seven-to-two that the Professional Golfers Association must allow Casey Martin, who has painful swelling of his right leg, to ride a cart while competing in tournaments. The Court noted that walking five miles or so around a golf course is not fundamental to the game and therefore Martin (with his serious physical impairment) merited that accommodation. (In his dissent, Justice Antonin Scalia called the majority's opinion a misguided intrusion of compassion into the rule of law—and the rules of golf—rather than a matter of justice.)

The ADA also addresses physical access within both new construction and existing structures. Provisions for new construction are straightforward. With few exceptions, new facilities must be "readily accessible to and useable by individuals with disabilities" (Title III, Sec. 303(a)(1)). Bowing to concerns about costs, the ADA does not require all new buildings with fewer than three stories or less than 3,000 square feet per story to install elevators. Health care settings carry stricter access standards: professional offices of health care providers cannot claim this exemption and must install an elevator, as must shopping centers (Sec. 303(b)).

Specifying ADA accessibility requirements for existing structures sparked heated Congressional debate. Expecting high costs and structural difficulties to retrofitting old buildings, businesses lobbied aggressively against initial drafts of the legislation. To avoid defeat, ADA supporters had to substantially rewrite the language:

> The original bill, S. 2345, required that nearly every place of public accommodation had to remove all barriers within five years. This provision earned S. 2345 the nickname of the "flat earth" bill. Drafters of S. 933, however, dispensed with the idea of wholesale retrofitting. Instead they required that all *new* construction be accessible. Nevertheless, they did not want to leave existing structures untouched. Consequently, drafters created a new legal term. S. 933 required that businesses make changes to existing structures where accessibility was "readily achievable." (Young, 1997, 101)

The ADA defines readily achievable renovations as changes that are structurally feasible and not too expensive. As shown in Table 9.3, ADA regulations list examples of steps to remove barriers that are generally considered readily achievable. Some changes, such as repositioning paper towel and cup dispensers and installing raised toilet seats, cost little. Others, such as widening doorways, repositioning toilet partitions, and installing new carpeting, may cost hundreds or thousands of dollars depending on what remodeling and structural changes are required.

Table 9.3
Examples of Steps to Remove Barriers

ADA Title III Regulations, 28 CFR Part 36, Sec. 36.304(b)

  (1) Installing ramps;
  (2) Making curb cuts in sidewalks and entrances;
  (3) Repositioning shelves;
  (4) Rearranging tables, chairs, vending machines, display racks, and other furniture;
  (5) Repositioning telephones;
  (6) Adding raised markings on elevator control buttons;
  (7) Installing flashing alarm lights;
  (8) Widening doors;
  (9) Installing offset hinges to widen doorways;
(10) Eliminating a turnstile or providing an alternative accessible path;
(11) Installing accessible door hardware;
(12) Installing grab bars in toilet stalls;
(13) Rearranging toilet partitions to increase maneuvering space;
(14) Insulating lavatory pipes under sinks to prevent burns;
(15) Installing a raised toilet seat;
(16) Installing a full-length bathroom mirror;
(17) Repositioning the paper towel dispenser in a bathroom;
(18) Creating designated accessible parking spaces;
(19) Installing an accessible paper cup dispenser at an existing inaccessible water fountain;
(20) Removing high pile, low density carpeting; or
(21) Installing vehicle hand controls.

As a concession to political and practical realities, the ADA explicitly acknowledges that accessibility sometimes cannot be readily achieved. In these instances, providers must offer goods or services to persons with disabilities "through alternative methods, if those methods are readily achievable" (28 CFR Part 36, Sec. 36.305(a)). Alternatives to barrier removal include "(1) Providing curb services or home delivery; (2) Retrieving merchandise from inaccessible shelves or racks; (3) Relocating activities to accessible locations" (28 CFR Part 36, Sec. 36.305(b)). Thus, the ADA leaves loopholes for people like Joe Alto to address.

INCOME SUPPORT PROGRAMS FOR PERSONS WITH DISABILITIES

Persons with MS often must stop working because of progressive disability or other problems, such as extreme fatigue. In 2005, we conducted a telephone survey of 983 working-age persons with MS living in communities nationwide, and we found that only 40 percent were working for pay (Iezzoni and Ngo, 2007). Half (50 percent) said they were not working because of their health, and 10 percent reported not working for some other reason. Some of these unemployed persons had spouses who were working, generating sufficient income to pay the family's bills. Others, like Joe Alto, needed income support from public (governmental) programs.

The Social Security Act authorizes two programs that provide cash benefits and health insurance eligibility to persons with disabilities:

- Social Security Disability Insurance (SSDI, under Title II of the Social Security Act); and
- Supplemental Security Income (SSI, under Title XVI).

SSDI gives benefits to persons who are considered insured by virtue of having worked and contributed to the Social Security Trust Fund through withholdings on their earnings. SSDI also covers certain disabled dependents of insured persons. The 1972 amendments to the Social Security Act granted eligibility for Medicare—the federal health insurance program for persons who are age 65 and older—to people who have received SSDI cash benefits for two years.

Title XVI provides SSI payments to persons, including children, who are disabled, blind, or elderly and have passed a so-called means test that documents low income and limited assets. Persons qualifying for SSI immediately receive Medicaid coverage—the joint federal-state health insurance program for persons who are poor and meet other categorical requirements. Some states supplement the federal benefit with additional cash payments. Poor persons receiving SSDI can also obtain SSI benefits after passing the means test.

People can also purchase long-term disability insurance from their employers. These private policies might not be available to all workers: part-time employees are often excluded from eligibility for benefits such as long-term disability insurance, and persons previously diagnosed with MS might face difficulties obtaining coverage. Different private long-term disability insurance policies have varying requirements and restrictions. Private long-term disability insurance policies provide monthly cash payments at prespecified levels (sometimes based on a percentage of the employee's salary), depending on the amount of insurance purchased.

The United States was the last major industrial nation to enact public income support (Stone, 1984). While the Social Security Act of 1935 covered elderly people, federal disability insurance arrived over two decades later. Anxious to prevent abuses, Congress structured Social Security as the last resort for people who could not work because of long-term, medically proven impairments. SSDI and SSI use identical definitions of disability for adult participants (see Table 9.4). To qualify, working-age persons must meet a yes/no standard: either they can or cannot engage in substantial gainful activity (work for which persons can be paid) because of medically proven physical or mental impairments.

To assess claims for disability insurance, the Social Security Administration contracts with each state's Disability Determination Service to assess the medical merit of applicants. States start their determination process by examining a Listing of Impairments, which itemizes impairments, grouped by body system and diseases, that should be sufficiently severe to preclude substantial gainful employment among adults. For MS, the Listing identifies three items:

- Significant and persistent disorganization of motor function in two extremities, resulting in sustained disturbance of gross and dexterous movements or gait and station
- Visual or mental impairments
- Significant, reproducible fatigue of motor function with substantial muscle weakness on repetitive activity (Social Security Administration, 2008)

One challenge to persons with MS in meeting Social Security eligibility standards is the waxing and waning course of the disease. Especially for individuals

Table 9.4
Social Security Disability Definitions

Definition of Disability
"For all individuals applying for disability benefits under title II, and for adults applying under title XVI, the definition of disability is the same. The law defines disability as the inability to engage in any substantial gainful activity (SGA) by reason of any medically determinable physical or mental impairment(s) which can be expected to result in death or which has lasted or can be expected to last for a continuous period of not less than 12 months." (Social Security Administration, 2008)

Medically Determinable Impairment
" . . . an impairment that results from anatomical, physiological, or psychological abnormalities which can be shown by medically acceptable clinical and laboratory diagnostic techniques. A physical or mental impairment must be established by medical evidence consisting of signs, symptoms, and laboratory findings—not only by the individual's statement of symptoms." (Social Security Administration, 2008)

with relapsing-remitting MS, they may not exhibit the sustained impairments required by Social Security. However, once the disease progresses to the point that persons need constant support from mobility aids, the likelihood of qualifying for SSDI or SSI is generally high—so long as persons have detailed documentation of their physical impairments from their neurologists.

In our survey of 983 working-age persons with MS living in the community, we found the following (Iezzoni and Ngo, 2007):

- 28 percent had SSDI only.
- 4 percent had SSI only.
- 5 percent had both SSDI and SSI.
- 29 percent had long-term private disability insurance, but 62 percent of these persons had obtained this insurance before being diagnosed with MS.
- 23 percent had Medicare as their only health insurance.
- 4 percent had Medicaid as their only health insurance.
- 4 percent had both Medicare and Medicaid health insurance.
- 74 percent had private health insurance, 84 percent of these through an employer or former employer.

Although most of the 983 survey respondents did not report significant stresses relating to money, a worrisome percentage did. Approximately 16 percent reported considerable difficulty paying for health care; 27 percent had put off or postponed seeking needed health care because of costs; 22 percent had delayed filling prescriptions, skipped medication doses, or split pills because of costs; and 27 percent reported considerable worries about affording basic necessities, such as food, utilities, and housing. For these individuals, financial stresses compound the anxieties that likely already accompany their MS.

PUBLIC TRANSPORTATION

Title II, Subtitle B of the ADA mandates that public transportation must be "readily accessible to and usable by individuals with disabilities, including individuals who use wheelchairs" (Section 222(a)). Accessible public transportation, with its promise of independence and easy movement, had been at the forefront of the disability rights agenda in the 1980s. Transportation issues differ by region, depending on whether goals involve retrofitting old systems (as in New York City and Boston) or building new networks (as in the San Francisco Bay Area and Washington, D.C.). Transportation systems reflect regional terrains, decades-old policy decisions, and shifting population patterns.

Depending on local factors, public transportation for people with disabilities generally gravitates toward either services separate from the main public systems (so-called paratransit) or integrated systems accessible to all. Some areas, especially rural and isolated regions, may have little or no accessible transportation at all. Metropolitan Boston melds these two approaches through accessible public buses on all fixed routes, accessible subways and trains, and a so-called demand response system, The RIDE. Intentions do not always match reality: essential accessibility equipment—such as wheelchair lifts on public buses, ramps on certain trolley cars, and elevators at subway stations—often malfunction.

With fleets of large vans with automatic wheelchair lifts, The RIDE serves people who cannot manage the fixed route systems alone or who need to go someplace accessible buses, subways, and trains do not reach. To qualify for The RIDE, persons must pass a medical determination, based on information provided by their doctors. Persons disabled by MS, such as Joe Alto, have no difficulty qualifying. For efficiency, RIDE vans often load multiple passengers simultaneously, meaning that riders sometimes take numerous detours before reaching their final destinations. RIDE users who have time for such delays tolerate the inconvenience, balanced against very low fares and reasonable accessibility. But others find themselves frequently frustrated, wasting their time, and showing up late for critical appointments.

EMPLOYMENT AND WORKPLACE ACCOMMODATIONS

Title I of the ADA bars discrimination against persons with disabilities in employment—hiring and firing, advancement, compensation, training, and benefits. The law applies to businesses with at least 15 employees, requiring employers to provide reasonable accommodations that do not cause them undue hardship (significant difficulties or expenses or fundamental redefinitions of jobs). Among reasonable accommodations the ADA includes ensuring physical access, restructuring jobs or work schedules, adjusting training activities and materials, acquiring or modifying assistive devices, and reassigning people to other jobs within the organization.

Reasonable accommodations vary according to the nature of the underlying medical problem. Progressive chronic conditions that wax and wane, relapse and remit (such as MS) pose different challenges than problems with fixed functional deficits (such as an amputation or spinal cord injury). During a flare, a person with MS may have to reduce work activities both to rest and to visit his or her neurologist. Flexible schedules can substantially improve the ability of people with MS or other chronic conditions to continue working.

The Job Accommodation Network (JAN) is a Web site sponsored by the U.S. Department of Labor's Office of Disability Employment Policy (www.jan.wvu.edu).

JAN consults with employers to give advice about hiring, retention, and promotion of persons with disabilities, as well as designing reasonable accommodations that suit both employee and employer. For persons with disabilities, JAN provides education about their employment rights under the ADA and assists with identifying accommodation strategies. JAN staff can provide individual work-site technical assistance services. The JAN Internet Web site contains more than 300 disability-specific accommodation publications.

JAN's Searchable Online Accommodation Resource (SOAR) has a specific link relating to MS. The SOAR MS Web site categorizes accommodation resources and strategies according to the nature of an individual's specific problem, including the following groupings for MS:

- Fatigue and weakness
- Cognitive limitations
- Fine motor limitations (difficulties with fingers and hands)
- Gross motor limitations (such as problems with walking)
- Sensitivity to extreme temperatures
- Vision impairment

Despite the ADA, some employers are better than others in proactively offering accommodations to their employees with MS. As Joe Alto said, people need to know their rights. Fifteen years before the ADA's passage, Sally Ann Jones (see Chapter 2) worked for a state university, which accommodated her needs beautifully. "I worked in an old building," Mrs. Jones recalled. In the morning,

the parking lot would fill up with cars. I made them designate a parking spot for me so I wouldn't have to walk so far. They did that cheerfully, although no one else—even the Dean—had a designated parking spot.

The first year I worked there, my office was on the second floor, and the women's toilet was on the first floor—no elevator. One day I said they had to reverse the toilet on the second floor from a men's room to a women's room, which they did in a second and didn't complain about it. The building had half a dozen stairs at the front, but there was no handrail. I went to the Dean and told him to put a handrail up: I have to haul myself up these stairs. So they did that for me. Then, my doctor insisted I had to have an air-conditioned office, so they bought a little air conditioner. I was the only person with air conditioning, so everybody was in my office all the time! And the last thing was, I couldn't do the stairs to the second floor anymore. It was too draining. So they moved my office to the first floor and switched the bathroom back again.

Gerald Bernadine, a businessman, had a radically different experience with his employer after the ADA (Iezzoni, 2003). "I started to trip while walking to work," recounted Mr. Bernadine. "Towards the end of the day, I couldn't lift my legs up to the next stair." After tests confirmed his MS diagnosis, Mr. Bernadine told his employer. At first, his employer responded well.

> They said, "Gerald, we're going to do whatever you need. If you need to go home, just let us know. Any problems, anything we can do to make it easier for you, just let us know." That all sounded great. I went back to my work with renewed energy, positive attitude. And what happened over those next six months was that they kept piling more and more work on me. No accommodations. They made me supervise four floors of office space in another building downtown. That wasn't even in my job description. They were not doing things to make it easier.

With his increasing walking difficulties, these additional responsibilities overwhelmed Mr. Bernadine.

"I was going to try to sort things out," Mr. Bernadine said, "and then they fired me. They waited until after Christmas, because you don't fire anybody at Christmas time. They called me one Monday morning after the holiday and told me it wasn't working out and that I was fired." Mr. Bernadine found a lawyer and sued the firm for failure to provide reasonable accommodations. In court, his employers argued that their company was in such financial distress that they could not offer reasonable accommodations to Mr. Bernadine. But the jury did not buy the employer's defense. His accommodation requests had required minimal, if any, expenditures from the company.

The company had offered Mr. Bernadine $3 million to settle his disability discrimination case, but he refused on principle. Although the court eventually awarded him about two-thirds of that amount, Mr. Bernadine felt vindicated, that he had proven his point: disabled people have rights. When asked how employers view hiring people with disabilities, Mr. Bernadine responded, "Employers are being dragged to the altar. It's a shotgun wedding. They're resisting. It just hasn't registered."

AT HOME WITH FAMILY

Finally, the most intimate layer of the onion—the layer that wraps most closely around the person with MS—is the family. As shown in Table 9.1, compared with the general U.S. population, persons with MS are more likely to be married: 67 percent compared with 57 percent. They are also more likely to be divorced or separated: 18 percent compared with 11 percent. But only 18 percent of persons with MS live alone, compared with 26 percent in the general population.

According to the Sonya Slifka study, approximately 1 percent of persons with MS live in assisted living facilities or nursing homes (Minden et al., 2006). Others, even with serious mobility impairments, remain in their homes—and with their families. They make accommodations for themselves. The vast majority of people with MS do not need intensive assistance in their homes, although they may—as does Sally Ann Jones, now a widow—need some personal help with errands and housekeeping.

Meeting daily needs can demand calculated logistics: every aspect of life is planned. Fears can creep in—of falling or of being immobilized, trapped in a fire, burned while cooking, or alone. People parse precious energy carefully. "I got stuck in the bathtub once," said one woman.

> With MS you can't afford to get overheated. I was in that shower and it felt so good. But by the time I got ready to get out of the bathtub, I couldn't move my legs. Nobody was home. I stayed in the bathtub with the water running for two-and-a-half hours. Then my son comes and asks, "What are you doing in the tub like that?" I had one leg half out and half in. I will never take a hot shower again.

Most private homes and smaller apartment buildings have numerous barriers, which are dangerous for persons with disabilities. Examples include stairs, insubstantial handrails, narrow doorways and halls (which impede wheelchair and walker passage), inadequate supports at critical locations (such as absent grab bars near toilets and in showers), and cramped bathrooms. As Mr. Goodall put it, his house offers vertical living while he prefers horizontal.

Most existing private properties predate federal and state accessibility laws. An early draft of the ADA included housing provisions, but this section was dropped and inserted into the Fair Housing Amendments Act of 1988. These amendments added people with disabilities as a group protected from discrimination in private housing to the Fair Housing Act, representing the first time antidiscrimination provisions for people with disabilities extended to the private sector. The 1988 amendments prohibit homeowners from refusing to rent or sell housing to someone because of disability or to charge them higher rents, sales prices, or security deposits. In addition, the law mandates physical accessibility of new construction of multifamily dwellings with four or more units and ensures that disabled people can adapt their residences to meet their needs.

Renovations are costly, however, and generally people must pay for these alterations themselves. Before his death, Sally Ann Jones and her husband widened doorways, installed ramps, and built a shower without a threshold so that she can roll into it unimpeded. Sometimes costly changes don't work. One woman with MS replaced her plush wall-to-wall carpets at great expense with highly polished hardwood floors, which she thought were not only elegant but would also be easier when using walkers and wheelchairs (which is true). But one day while playing cards with her mother and sitting in a chair with rolling casters, the chair slipped on the waxed surface and spilled her onto the floor. The fall fractured her hip. She wonders how to tell her husband, a policeman with a modest income, that she wants to reinstall carpets.

The most common home adaptation is installing grab bars or special railings, followed by ramps, making extra-wide doors, and raised toilet seats. To be safe and secure, grab bars must be screwed or nailed firmly into sturdy supports. Many people use plastic shower chairs when it becomes unsafe to stand. Other strategies can improve independence and safety at home. People carry small cell phones in their pockets so they can reach help in emergencies. So-called lifeline services summon emergency assistance when the person presses the button of a pendant worn around his or her neck. People rearrange household items for furniture surfing—placing objects strategically to grab for balance. Every chair and table is perfectly positioned to provide support.

Oftentimes, environmental adaptations are not enough, and people need human help with daily activities. The dynamics of who provides this assistance —and its effects on interpersonal relationships—are complicated. Some people hire professional personal care assistants, home health aides, housekeepers, Meals on Wheels, grocery delivery services, or other services among the expanding industry aimed at facilitating independent living at home. But most people turn first to family. Of course, the majority of individuals don't want to burden their spouses, partners, or children, but they also don't want to leave home or to go into a nursing home. Some feel uncomfortable having strangers assist with meeting daily needs. So family members help out.

This help carries many nuances and consequences for the disabled person and caregiver, over time. As psychiatrist and anthropologist Arthur Kleinman (1988, 45) observed about the mundane, daily demands of chronic illness, "There is a kind of quiet heroism that comes from meeting these problems and the sentiments they provoke, of getting through the long course with grace and spirit and even humor; sick persons and their families understand the courage." But many people reject this notion of heroism, asking, "What else can you do but get through?"

Gerald Bernadine recognized that his MS not only redefined his self-perceptions to some extent, but also shaped his interactions with others, sometimes in unanticipated ways. "Part of getting on with your life is acceptance," Mr. Bernadine observed.

> If you don't accept it, if you deny it, that's probably the worst thing you could do. It seems like the people that get disabled are the people that have always been self-sufficient, self-reliant, the person out front. Wait a second —bingo! They get pulled down with a disability. I was used to being very self-reliant, independent. And so, when I got MS, I finally just had to accept that I was ill. I had to accept limitations. I had to accept a helping hand from people. One thing that I've learned is that, when somebody reaches out to help you—even if you don't need that help—it's really nice to accept it. Because it does something for them, too. It creates that bond which is really special. I think they get as much out of it as I do.

Nancy Mairs (1996, 73–74), an author with MS, has known her husband George for 35 years.

> After so many years together, we tend to communicate telegraphically. . . . At the mundane level, where most of my needs for assistance reside, we carry out our tasks almost without comment. . . .
> This almost intuitive communication, which can evolve between people who live in intimacy and affection over a long span, offers inexpressible comfort, and in our precarious circumstances, both of us want comforting more than most. He tells me he is no more eager to relinquish his caregiving role—which he finds "seductive, because the world esteems me for it"—than I am to hire outside assistance.

All marriages—and partnerships with significant others—are complicated works in progress. This is especially true for people with progressive chronic conditions. Mairs (1996, 74) and her husband recognize practical realities and the inevitability of change: "We both know that as my condition deteriorates, he can't take on the extra work without growing weary and grumpy." George has had malignant melanoma, the most lethal form of skin cancer. They anticipate seismic shifts in their daily lives, hopes, and expectations should his disease recur. Over the long haul, few marriages are truly one-sided.

Conventional wisdom holds that stresses caused by MS end marriages, especially tenuous ones. Three factors appear disruptive: partners' inability to share equally the MS illness experience, despite good intentions; compromised traditional gender roles; and emotions generated when partners become caretakers

(Leino-Kilpi, Luoto, and Katajisto, 1998). But a study of 125 persons with MS found that, although 55 percent of relationships with spouses changed after diagnosis, 49 percent of these changes were positive (Eklund and MacDonald, 1991). Another study of 100 people with MS found that people felt their health problems brought them closer to their spouses and allowed them more time together, especially if the partner with MS stopped working full time (Wassem, 1991).

When talking about dealing with disability, many people abandon the first person, singular pronoun—instead of I, they speak of we. They and their spouse or partner are in it together. While both cannot share the illness experience, they confront its consequences as a team. The shift in language is subtle, but the implications are profound. As recounted in Chapter 2, for Sally Ann Jones and her husband, this shift happened on the day of diagnosis.

"My husband came in and asked me what the doctor had said. I told him that I have MS, and my husband sort of sighed. Then he said, 'At least we know what it is. Now we can deal with it.'"

* * * * *

The kind neurologist who suspected that I had MS during my December 1980 visit (see the Preface) said something that became an essential fabric of my existence: that the course of MS is unpredictable, so I would have to live with uncertainty (Iezzoni, 2003). I could not know, until my life had passed, how it would all turn out. So, I might as well go ahead and live my life. This brave assertion belies the bewilderment I felt then. I was more shell-shocked, confused, and sad than angry. Once I started seeing patients in medical school, I daily confronted human tragedies wrought by diseases, physical and mental, and my own situation seemed comparatively minor. I could still walk, albeit with an unsteady, broadbased gait. As described in Chapter 8, I started using a cane only after a fall during my surgery clerkship. I completed the four years of medical school and graduated without pause. But, although I truly enjoyed interacting with patients, a constant sorrow shadowed me.

Confronting the physical limitations and uncertainty of MS was only one step. I also had to deal with people's reactions to me—the me they equated with my MS. A decade before the ADA, Harvard Medical School was a tough place to absorb these lessons. My neurologist warned me that my clinical training would have to be altered. I could not stay up all night in the hospital taking call: the risks of exacerbating the MS through long sleepless hours were too great. While I sought neither sympathy nor pity from the academic authorities, I had hoped for understanding and some gentleness. I soon learned that those qualities were in short supply. The medical school immediately assigned me to a new academic advisor, a psychiatrist. When I walked into his office for our initial advisory meeting, his words rushed out: "Don't expect me to be your friend. I'm here to give academic advice, not emotional support."

I never became a practicing physician. Early during my clinical training, I received explicit hints that my medical career was in jeopardy. On my first day in the operating room during my surgical rotation, the attending surgeon let me hold a finger retractor during a delicate procedure. Once the concentrated silence broke and closing the surgical wound began, the surgeon turned to me, "What's the worst part of your disease?"

Embarrassed by the assembled team of residents and nurses at the operating table, I demurred.

"Do you want my opinion?" the surgeon asked. The scrub nurse rolled her eyes at me sympathetically, and knowing I had no option, I nodded. "You will make a terrible doctor. You lack the most important quality in a good doctor— accessibility."

Late in my third year, I began thinking about applying for an internal medicine residency. At a student dinner, I sat next to a top leader at a Harvard teaching hospital and decided to ask his advice. I would not be able to stay up all night; perhaps I could share a residency with someone else. Few other accommodations seemed necessary. "What would your hospital think of my situation?" I asked.

"Frankly," he replied in a conversational tone, "there are too many doctors in the country right now for us to worry about training handicapped physicians. If that means certain people get left by the wayside, that's too bad."

Over the next months, after a wrenching internal debate (joined by my husband, caring but realistic), I decided not to battle for an internship but to go straight into research. From four years at medical school (long before confessional talk shows and social networking pages on the Internet), I left with one overwhelming lesson: never, ever, talk about IT, the MS! It can't be cured, so be silent. Don't mention it. For 15 years, I almost never did.

I can summarize quickly what happened after I graduated from medical school in 1984. I had trouble getting a job. Prospective employers raised my MS as either a reason not to hire me or to pay me only half a salary. I was hired only after a senior physician who had taken notice of me—and whose daughter also had MS—telephoned someone at a neighboring university and convinced him to hire me. Fortunately, work went well. I spent six years in that job before returning to Harvard Medical School as a faculty member. I found a small circle of wonderful, supportive colleagues.

I understand the realities underlying my career success. My husband, a hematologist and oncologist (blood and cancer doctor), does the chores around our house—the grocery shopping, the laundry, the yard work, the gardening, and the kitty litter—and I sit at my computer, writing and working (I still cook a little, although knives scare me). My husband's help allows me to concentrate on my work, at some cost to his own career. Time restored my spirit lost in the grey fog of diagnosis and medical school, although my subconscious mind remembers my walking past: I still awake occasionally from dreams of running.

Over time, I came to realize that silence about my MS carries consequences. Silence reinforces the stigmatization of disability, the sense of shame and guilt, that becoming disabled and unable to walk is something to hide—although, of course, we can't. Most importantly, strangers ask my advice. In my wheelchair, I have become a sort of rolling focus group, attracting unsolicited questions from strangers about themselves or their relatives with difficulties walking. Sometimes those family members or friends have MS. The strangers want advice about restoring mobility, keeping going, and reconnecting with the world. The stories of the many generous individuals who have spoken with me, such as Sally Ann Jones, Lester Goodall, Joni and Jenny, Gerald Bernadine, and Joe Alto, make clear that countless people with MS live daily with grit and grace. Their lives are rich and varied, and they keep on going. We can learn from them and from each other about living with MS.

Timeline

1380	Birth of Virgin Lidwina (1380–1433) in Schiedam, Holland. May be first documented case of MS
1794	Birth of Augustus d'Esté (1794–1848), grandson of King George III of England, who kept an extensive diary documenting probable MS symptoms
1824	First description by a physician, Frenchman Charles Prosper Ollivier d'Angers (1796–1845), of a likely MS case
1838	Scottish physician Robert Carswell (1793–1857) makes the first illustration of how MS damages nerves
1866	French physician-scientist Edmé Vulpian (1826–1887) first employs the phrase "sclérose en plaque disséminée"
1868	Parisian neurologist Jean-Martin Charcot (1825–1893) gives three lectures that present, for the first time, comprehensive clinical and pathological descriptions identifying MS as a disease
1878	Neurologist Edward Constant Seguin (1843–1898) of New York publishes reports on two cases of MS

1882	British physician Sir Byrom Bramwell (1847–1931) publishes a textbook on MS identifying injury as a potential cause
1884	French physician Pierre Marie (1853–1940) publishes an article linking MS with infectious diseases
1885	German physician Heinrich Irenaeus Quincke (1842–1922) develops therapeutic lumbar puncture
1897	Joseph-François-Félix Babinski (1857–1923), French physician, publishes an article about plantar reflex in MS (upgoing great toe upon stimulating lateral sole of foot)
1921	Meeting of MS experts rejects claim of American psycho-analyst Smith Ely Jelliffe (1866–1945) that repressed emotions cause MS
1924	Jacques Lhermitte (1877–1959), French neurologist, describes tingling, electrical sensation from flexing neck in MS
1942	New York neuroscientist Elvin A. Kabat (1914–2000) identifies immunoglobulin patterns in the cerebrospinal fluid (CSF) of persons with MS
1943–1960	MS epidemic occurs on the isolated Faroe Islands, a semi-independent territory of Denmark between Iceland and Norway
1945	Sylvia Lawry (1915–2001) places an advertisement in the *New York Times* asking anyone who has recovered from MS to contact her; her younger brother Bernard had MS
1948	Founding of National Multiple Sclerosis Society (NMSS) in the United States, spurred by the efforts of Sylvia Lawry (1915–2001)
1950	NMSS funds the first major study of MS in the United States and Canada
1950	Criteria to classify relapsing-remitting and progressive patterns of MS are specified
1951	Use of cortisone in treating MS
1955	American neurologist John F. Kurtzke outlines the Disability Status Scale

1957	Interferons are discovered
1961	Several researchers show that oligodendrocytes are responsible for myelination and remyelination
1962	NMSS cosponsors a conference on what causes demyelination
1964	Oligoclonal bands are demonstrated in CSF of patients with MS
1972	Evoked potential testing is applied to MS
1972	Relationship of MS to certain HLA types is identified
1974	CT scan finding of MS lesion is confirmed by biopsy
1977	Interferon beta-1a is developed
1981	First MRI scan of the brain occurs
1983	Kurtze specifies the Expanded Disability Status Scale
1988	Criteria are specified for identifying MS lesions using MRI
1993	FDA approves interferon beta-1b (Betaseron®)
1996	FDA approves interferon beta-1a (Avonex®) and glatiramer acetate (Copaxone®)
2000	FDA approves mitoxantrone (Novantrone®)
2002	FDA approves interferon beta-1a (Rebif®)
2004	FDA approves natalizumab (Tysabri®)
2005	FDA withdraws approval of natalizumab because of two deaths of patients from progressive multifocal leukoencephalopathy
2006	FDA reinstates approval of natalizumab use as a solo therapy

Glossary

Antibodies Proteins made by the body's immune system that bind to antigens or structures recognized as foreign to the body.

Antigen Material or structure recognized as foreign to the body and that can spur production of antibodies by the immune system.

Assistive technology Devices or equipment that compensate for functional impairments and allow persons with disabilities to perform various activities.

Ataxia Lack of coordination among muscles.

Autoimmune disease Condition in which the body's immune system malfunctions and attacks its own tissues or cells.

Axon Long process of a nerve cell that conducts impulses away from the cell body.

Blood-brain barrier Membrane that limits and controls passage of substances from the blood into the central nervous system.

Central nervous system Brain and spinal cord; oversees and coordinates all activities of the nervous system.

Cerebrospinal fluid Colorless liquid produced by filtering substances from the blood and by secretions from specialized brain cells; circulates around the brain and spinal cord, cushioning and protecting central nervous system tissues.

Demyelination Damage caused to the myelin sheath surrounding nerve axons.

Epidemiology Study of rates and patterns of disease occurrence within populations.

Flare Exacerbation or relapse, with new or worsening symptoms.

Glatiramer acetate Brand name Copaxone®; disease-modifying medication administered by daily subcutaneous injection.

Glucocorticoids Group of steroids involved in metabolism of carbohydrates, proteins, and fats that has anti-inflammatory and immunosuppressive abilities; used to treat acute flares or exacerbations of MS.

Human leukocyte antigen Proteins encoded by specific genes that appear on the surface of cells and are tolerated by the body's immune system.

Immune system Bodily system involving numerous cell types and complex chemical compounds that defend the body against foreign cells, substances, and other invaders; when it malfunctions, as in autoimmune diseases, it can also attack self.

Immunosuppression Suppression or reduction of immune system activity.

Inflammation Microscopic response to bodily injury marked by aggregation of various immune system cells that act to eliminate foreign substances and restore normal functioning.

Interferon Several different types of cytokines (chemical substances produced by immune system cells) that play various roles in regulating immune system responses.

Interferon beta Type of interferon produced by fibroblasts (connective tissue cell) that may reduce MS relapse rates; several different products are marketed under brand names Avonex®, Betaseron®, and Rebif® and require administration by injection on varying schedules.

Lesion Abnormal change in body structure or tissues caused by disease process or injury.

Magnetic resonance imaging Diagnostic scanning (imaging) technique that produces pictures of internal tissues by applying radio waves that cause atoms in tissues to respond; computers detect atomic level responses and compile them to generate detailed images.

Mitoxantrone Brand name Novantrone®; disease-modifying medication with possible heart toxicity; administered by intravenous infusion with limits in total dosages.

Motor functioning Movement of muscles, frequently abnormal in MS.

Multiple sclerosis (MS) Degenerative disease of the central nervous system caused by destruction of myelin sheaths and deterioration of nerve axons.

Myelin Whitish, fatty material laid down by oligodendrocytes around the axons of neurons within the central nervous system; myelin insulates axons and facilitates rapid conduction of nervous impulses.

Natalizumab Brand name Tysabri®; monoclonal antibody that may prevent activated immune cells from crossing the blood-brain barrier; associated with rare but lethal cases of progressive multifocal leukoencephalopathy.

Nerve Groups of neurons and specialized nerve cells that conduct and receive electrical impulses and govern bodily functions.

Neuroglia Supportive cells within the central nervous system.

Neurologist Doctor (physician) skilled in diagnosing and treating diseases of the nervous system.

Neurology Branch of medicine focused on functioning and diseases of the nervous system.

Neuron Nerve cell that receives or transmits signals within the nervous system.

Occupational therapy Rehabilitation approach that emphasizes assisting patients in performing activities of daily living using various strategies, including orthotics and assistive technologies.

Oligodendrocyte Cell in the central nervous system that produces myelin.

Optic neuritis Inflammation of the optic nerve, resulting in eye pain and vision loss.

Orthotic Mechanical support or brace for weak joints or muscles.

Pathology Anatomical and physiological deviations from normal that define or characterize particular diseases.

Physiatrist Doctor (physician) expert in physical medicine and rehabilitation.

Physical therapy Rehabilitation approach that aims to improve physical functioning or reduce impairments using various methods, such as exercise or using assistive technologies.

Plaque Areas where the myelin sheath surrounding axons has been damaged.

Primary progressive Second most common pattern of MS (about 10 percent of new diagnoses); symptoms slowly progress with no true remissions, although persons may sometimes experience periods during which symptoms and disability remain stable.

Progressive relapsing. Rarest form of newly diagnosed MS (5 percent). Insidious onset of neurological symptoms, with occasional periods of relapses and remissions overlaying slow progression.

Relapse Acute attack or exacerbation.

Relapsing-remitting Most common pattern of MS among newly diagnosed patients (about 85 percent); symptoms occur and then resolve after varying periods of time.

Remission Abatement or resolution of symptoms.

Secondary progressive MS pattern in which persons with relapsing-remitting MS gradually experience increasing disability or symptoms, without periods of remission; large percentage of persons with relapsing-remitting MS transition into secondary progressive MS, sometimes many years after being diagnosed.

Spasticity Involuntary contraction of muscles, causing spasms or stiffness.

Spinal cord Thick bundle of nerves and associated structures that extends from the brain down through the canal formed by the vertebrae and transmits and receives nervous system signals between the brain and nerves throughout the body; along with the brain, comprises the central nervous system.

T cells Immune system cells that develop in the thymus and might participate in myelin destruction in MS.

White matter Nerve tissues in the brain and spinal cord that are whitish in color and consist primarily of myelinated nerve fibers.

Internet Resources

Numerous Web sites address issues related to MS. Below are selected Web sites, which cover a range of topics. Appearance on this list does not constitute an endorsement of the accuracy or usefulness of information available on these Web sites. As always, persons should treat information taken from Web sites cautiously.

American Academy of Neurology
1080 Montreal Avenue
Saint Paul, MN 55116
http://www.aan.com/
Tel: 800-879-1960 or 651-695-2717
Fax: 651-695-2791
An international professional association of neurologists and neuroscience professionals. The Web site contains information about guidelines for caring for various neurological conditions, including MS.

American Academy of Physical Medicine and Rehabilitation
330 North Wabash Avenue, Suite 2500
Chicago, IL 60611-7617

http://www.aapmr.org/
Tel: 312-464-9700
Fax: 312-464-0227
The professional association of physical medicine and rehabilitation (PM&R) physicians (also known as physiatrists). The Web site contains information about the profession, practitioners throughout the United States, and training requirements.

The American Occupational Therapy Association, Inc.
4720 Montgomery Lane
P.O. Box 31220
Bethesda, MD 20824-1220
http://www.aota.org/
Tel: 301-652-2682
Fax: 301-652-7711
The national professional association of occupational therapists. The Web site contains information about occupational therapy services and training requirements.

American Physical Therapy Association
1111 North Fairfax Street
Alexandria, VA 22314-1488
http://www.apta.org
Tel: 800-999-APTA (2782)
703-684-APTA (2782)
TDD: 703-683-6748
Fax: 703-684-7343
The national professional association of physical therapists. The Web site contains information about physical therapy services and training requirements.

Consortium of Multiple Sclerosis Centers
359 Main Street, Suite A
Hackensack, NJ 07601
http://www.mscare.org/cmsc/index.php
Tel: 201-487-1050
Fax: 201-678-2290
Consortium of multidisciplinary centers (clinical programs involving different types of health care professionals) that specialize in providing care to persons with MS around the country.

Accelerated Cure Project for Multiple Sclerosis
300 Fifth Avenue
Waltham, MA 02451
http://www.acceleratedcure.org
Tel: 781-487-0008
Fax: 781-487-0009
Nonprofit organization dedicated to curing MS by understanding its causes; focuses on developing a blood, tissue, and data bank.

DisabilityInfo.gov
http://www.disabilityinfo.gov
1-800-FED-INFO (1-800-333-4636/voice and TTY)
Online resource produced by the federal government and designed to provide access to disability-related information and programs available across the government, including benefits, civil rights, community life, education, employment, housing, health, technology, and transportation.

Job Accommodation Network
P.O. Box 6080
Morgantown, WV 26506-6080
http://www.jan.wvu.edu/
Tel: 800-526-7234 (V) in the United States
800-ADA-WORK [800-232-9675] (V) in the United States
877-781-9403 (TTY) in the United States
304-293-7186 (V) locally and outside the United States
Fax: 304-293-5407
Service provided by the U.S. Department of Labor's Office of Disability Employment Policy that supports the employment, including self-employment and small business ownership, of people with disabilities

Multiple Sclerosis Association of America
706 Haddonfield Road
Cherry Hill, NJ 08002
http://www.msassociation.org
Tel: 856-488-4500 or 800-532-7667
Fax: 856-661-9797
National, nonprofit organization that provides support and direct services to individuals with MS and their families.

Multiple Sclerosis Foundation
6350 North Andrews Avenue
Ft. Lauderdale, FL 33309-2130
http://www.msfocus.org
Tel: 954-776-6805 888-MSFOCUS (673-6287)
Fax: 954-351-0630
Nonprofit organization that provides national toll-free telephone support, educational programs, homecare services, support groups, assistive technology programs, and educational publications, among other programs.

National Multiple Sclerosis Society
733 Third Avenue
3rd Floor
New York, NY 10017-3288
http://www.nationalmssociety.org
Tel: 212-986-3240 800-344-4867 (FIGHTMS)
Fax: 212-986-7981
National nonprofit organization that funds MS research, provides extensive educational and informational services, helps with employment issues, offers free counseling, runs self-help groups, advocates for people with disabilities, and provides referrals to medical professionals.

National Institute of Allergy and Infectious Diseases, National Institutes of Health
NIAID Office of Communications and Government Relations
6610 Rockledge Drive, MSC 6612
Bethesda, MD 20892-6612
http://www3.niaid.nih.gov/topics/autoimmune/
Toll-Free: 866-284-4107
TDD: 800-877-8339 (for hearing impaired)
Fax: 301-402-3573
Online informational resource concerning autoimmunity and autoimmune diseases.

National Institute of Neurological Disorders and Stroke, National Institutes of Health
NIH Neurological Institute
P.O. Box 5801
Bethesda, MD 20824

Voice: 800-352-9424 or 301-496-5751
TTY (for people using adaptive equipment): 301-468-5981
http://www.ninds.nih.gov/disorders/multiple_sclerosis/multiple_sclerosis.htm
Online informational resource concerning MS.

New York Times
Times Health Guide: Multiple Sclerosis
http://health.nytimes.com/health/guides/disease/multiple-sclerosis/
overview.html
Information for consumers on issues related to MS drawn from *New York Times*
health reporting.

PatientsLikeMe™
Multiple Sclerosis Community
http://www.patientslikeme.com/multiple-sclerosis/community
Online, virtual community of >13,000 persons with MS who voluntarily enter
information about themselves and their MS symptoms and treatments into an
Internet-based database. Participants can compare their MS experiences with
those of other PatientsLikeMe members. Another goal is compiling findings from
all participants to learn more about MS and its treatments.

U.S. Department of Justice, Civil Rights Division, Disability Rights Section
U.S. Department of Justice
950 Pennsylvania Avenue, NW
Civil Rights Division
Disability Rights Section - NYA
Washington, D.C. 20530
Tel: 800-514-0301 (voice)
800-514-0383 (TTY)
Fax: 202-307-1198
http://www.usdoj.gov/crt/drs/drshome.php
Information about federal activities implementing and overseeing the Americans
with Disabilities Act (ADA). The Web site contains information about lawsuits
and actions brought by the federal government under the ADA, as well as infor-
mation for consumers about their rights under the law.

Bibliography

Ascherio, A., and K. Munger. "Epidemiology of Multiple Sclerosis: From Risk Factors to Prevention," *Seminars in Neurology* 28 (2008): 17–28.

Bar-Or, A. "Human Immune Studies in Multiple Sclerosis." In *Multiple Sclerosis and Demyelinating Diseases*. Edited by M. S. Freedman, 91–109. Philadelphia: Lippincott Williams & Wilkins, 2006.

Birnbaum, G. "Making the Diagnosis of Multiple Sclerosis." In *Multiple Sclerosis and Demyelinating Diseases*. Edited by M. S. Freedman, 11–124. Philadelphia: Lippincott Williams & Wilkins. 2006.

Chaudhuri, A., and P. O. Behan. "Multiple Sclerosis Is Not an Autoimmune Disease." *Archives of Neurology* 6 (2004): 1610–1612.

Compston, A., and A. Coles. "Multiple Sclerosis." *Lancet* 359 (2002): 1221–1231.

Compston, A., and C. Confavreux. "The Distribution of Multiple Sclerosis." In *McAlpine's Multiple Sclerosis*. 4th ed. Edited by A. Compston, C. Confavreux, H. Lassmann, I. McDonald, D. Miller, J. Noseworthy, K. Smith, and H. Wekerle, 71–111. Philadelphia: Churchill, Livingstone, Elsevier, 2005.

Compston, A., H. Lasserman, and I. McDonald. "The Story of Multiple Sclerosis." In *McAlpine's Multiple Sclerosis*. 4th ed. Edited by A. Compston, C. Confavreux, H. Lassmann, I. McDonald, D. Miller, J. Noseworthy, K. Smith, and H. Wekerle, 3–68. Philadelphia: Churchill, Livingstone, Elsevier, 2005.

Compston, A., H. Lassmann, and K. Smith. "The Neurobiology of Multiple Sclerosis." In *McAlpine's Multiple Sclerosis*. 4th ed. Edited by A. Compston, C. Confavreux, H. Lassmann, I. McDonald, D. Miller, J. Noseworthy, K. Smith, and H. Wekerle, 449–490. Philadelphia: Churchill, Livingston, Elsevier, 2005.

Eklund, V. A., and M. L. MacDonald. "Descriptions of Persons with Multiple Sclerosis with an Emphasis on What Is Needed from Psychologists." *Professional Psychology: Research and Practice* 22 (1991): 277–284.

Figg, L., and J. Farrell-Beck. "Amputation in the Civil War: Physical and Social Dimensions." *Journal of the History of Medicine and Allied Sciences* 48 (1993): 54–75.

Fleischer, D. Z., and F. Zames. *The Disability Rights Movement. From Charity to Confrontation*. Philadelphia: Temple University Press, 2001.

Gallagher, H. G. *Black Bird Fly Away: Disabled in an Able-Bodied World*. Arlington, VA: Vandamere Press, 1998.

———. *FDR's Splendid Deception*. Arlington, VA: Vandamere Press, 1994.

Hockenberry, J. *Moving Violations: War Zones, Wheelchairs, and Declarations of Independence*. New York: Hyperion, 1995.

Hoover, J. A. "Diversional Occupational Therapy in World War I: A Need for Purpose in Occupations." *American Journal of Occupational Therapy* 50 (1996): 881–885.

Iezzoni, L. I. *When Walking Fails. Mobility Problems of Adults with Chronic Conditions*. Berkeley: University of California Press, 2003.

Iezzoni, L. I., and L. Ngo. "Health, Disability, and Life Insurance Experiences of Working-Age Persons with Multiple Sclerosis." *Multiple Sclerosis* 13 (2007): 534–546.

Iezzoni, L. I., and B. L. O'Day. *More Than Ramps. A Guide to Improving Health Care Quality and Access for People with Disabilities*. New York: Oxford University Press, 2006.

Iezzoni, L. I., S. R. Rao, and R. P. Kinkel. "Patterns of Mobility Aid Use among Working-Age Persons with Multiple Sclerosis Living in the Community in the United States." *Disability and Health Journal* 2 (2009): 67–76.

Illingworth, P., and W. E. Parmet. "Positively Disabled. The Relationship between the Definition of Disability and Rights under the American Disability Act." In *Americans with Disabilities: Exploring Implications of the Law for Individuals and Institutions*. Edited by L. P. Francis and A. Silvers, 3–17. New York: Routledge, 2000.

Kamenetz, H. L. *The Wheelchair Book: Mobility for the Disabled*. Springfield, IL: Charles C. Thomas, 1969.

Karp, G. *Choosing a Wheelchair: A Guide for Optimal Independence*. Sebastopol, CA: O'Reilley and Associates, 1998.

Kiernan, J. A. *Barr's the Human Nervous System: An Anatomical Viewpoint*. 9th ed. Philadelphia: Lippincott Williams, & Wilkins; Wolters Kluwer, 2009.

Kleinman, A. *The Illness Narrative*. New York: Basic Books, 1988.

Kraft, G. H., and J. Y. Cui. "Multiple Sclerosis." In *Physical Medicine and Rehabilitation*. 4th ed. Edited by J. A. DeLisa and B. M. Gans. 1753–1769. Philadelphia: Lippincott Williams & Wilkins, 2005.

Kurtzke, J. F. "Epidemiology of Multiple Sclerosis. Does This Really Point Toward and Etiology?" Lectio Doctoralis. *Neurological Science* 21 (2000): 383–403.

Leino-Kilpi, H., E. Luoto, and J. Katajisto. "Elements of Empowerment and MS Patients." *The Journal of Neuroscience Nursing: Journal of the American Association of Neuroscience Nurses* 30 (1998): 116–123.

Linton, S. *Claiming Disability: Knowledge and Identity.* New York: New York University Press, 1998.

Lipton, H. L., Z. Liang, S. Hertzler, and K. N. Son. "A Specific Viral Cause of Multiple Sclerosis: One Virus, One Disease." *Annals of Neurology* 61 (2007): 514–523.

Mairs, N. *Waist High in the World. A Life Among the Nondisabled.* Boston: Beacon Press, 1996.

McDonald, I., and A. Compston. "The Symptoms and Signs of Multiple Sclerosis." In *McAlpine's Multiple Sclerosis.* 4th ed. Edited by A. Compston, C. Confavreux, H. Lassmann, I. McDonald, D. Miller, J. Noseworthy, K. Smith, and H. Wekerle, 287–346. Philadelphia: Churchill, Livingstone, Elsevier, 2005.

Minden, S. L., D. Frankel, L. Hadden, J. Perloffp, K. P. Srinath, and D. C. Hoaglin. "The Sonya Slifka Longitudinal Multiple Sclerosis Study: Methods and Sample Characteristics." *Multiple Sclerosis* 12 (2006): 24–38.

Moore, H. W. "Early Treatment for MS—Is It Worth It?" *Neurology Reviews.Com* 10, no. 1 (January 2002), www.neurologyreviews.com/nr/jan02/ms.html.

Morales, Y., J. E. Parisi, and C. F. Lucchinetti. The Pathology of Multiple Sclerosis. In *Multiple Sclerosis and Demyelinating Diseases..* Edited by M. S. Freedman, 27–45. Philadelphia: Lippincott Williams & Wilkins. 2006.

Murray, T. J. *Multiple Sclerosis: The History of a Disease.* New York: Demos, 2005.

National Center for Complementary and Alternative Medicine. "Health Topics A–Z." National Institutes of Health. www.nccam.nih.gov/ (accessed July 4, 2009).

National Institute of Neurological Diseases and Stroke (NINDS), "Multiple Sclerosis: Hope through Research." National Institutes of Health. www.ninds.nih.gov/disorders/multiple_sclerosis/detail_multiple_sclerosis.htm (accessed July 23, 2009).

National Institutes of Health, National Institute of Allergy and Infectious Diseases (NIAID), *Understanding the Immune System. How It Works.* NIH Publication No. 07-5423, 2007.

National Multiple Sclerosis Society. "Medications Used in MS." National Multiple Sclerosis Society, www.nationalmssociety.org/about-multiple-sclerosis/treatments/medications/index.aspx.

Olek, M. J. "Comorbid Problems Associated with Multiple Sclerosis in Adults." *UptoDate* Version 16.3. (October 14, 2008a), www.uptodate.com.

———. "Diagnosis of Multiple Sclerosis in Adults." *UptoDate* Version 16.3 (October 1, 2008b), www.uptodate.com.

———. "Epidemiology, Risk Factors, and Clinical Features of Multiple Sclerosis in Adults." *UptoDate* Version 16.3. (October 4, 2008c), www.uptodate.com.

———. "Treatment of Acute Exacerbations of Multiple Sclerosis in Adults." *UptoDate* Version 16.3. (October 1, 2008d), www.uptodate.com.

———. "Treatment of Progressive Multiple Sclerosis in Adults." *UptoDate* Version 16.3. (October 6, 2008e), www.uptodate.com.

———. "Treatment of Relapsing-Remitting Multiple Sclerosis in Adults." *UptoDate* Version 16.3. (October 16, 2008f), www.uptodate.com.

Olkin, R. *What Psychotherapists Should Know About Disability.* New York: The Guildford Press, 1999.

Pugliatti, M., G. Rosati, H. Carton, T. Riise, J. Drulovic, L. Vécsei, and I. Milanov. "The Epidemiology of Multiple Sclerosis in Europe." *European Journal of Neurology* 13 (2006): 700–722.

Sadovnick, A. D. "The Genetics and Genetic Epidemiology of Multiple Sclerosis." In *Multiple Sclerosis and Demyelinating Diseases.* Edited by M. S. Freedman, 17–25. Philadelphia: Lippincott Williams & Wilkins, 2006.

Shapiro, J. P. *No Pity: People with Disabilities Forging a New Civil Rights Movement.* New York: Times Books, 1994.

Sibley, W. A., C. R. Bamford, and K. Clark. "Clinical Viral Infections and Multiple Sclerosis." *Lancet* 1 (1985): 1313–1315.

Social Security Administration. "Disability Evaluation under Social Security" SSA pub. no.-64-039 in Social Security Administration [database online]. Washington, D.C., 2008. www.ssa.gov/disability/professionals/bluebook/11.00-Neurological-Adult .htm#Top.

Starr, P. *The Social Transformation of American Medicine: The Rise of a Sovereign Profession and the Making of a Vast Industry.* New York: Basic Books, Inc., 1982.

Stevenson, V. L., and E. D. Playford. "Rehabilitation and MS." *International MS Journal* 14 (2007): 85–92.

Stone, D. A. *The Disabled State.* Philadelphia: Temple University Press, 1984.

Toombs, S. K. "Sufficient unto the Day: A Life with Multiple Sclerosis." In *Chronic Illness: From Experience to Policy.* Edited by S. K. Toombs, D. Barnard, and R. D. Carson, 3–23. Bloomington: Indiana University Press, 1995.

U.S. Department of Labor, Bureau of Labor Statistics. *Occupational Outlook Handbook.* (2008–2009 Edition). U.S. Department of Labor. www.bls.gov/oco/ocos080.htm.

Wassem, R. "A Test of the Relationship between Health Locus of Control and the Course of Multiple Sclerosis." *Rehabilitation Nursing* 16 (1991): 189–193.

Young, J. M. Equality of Opportunity: The Making of the Americans with Disabilities Act. Washington, DC: National Council on Disability, 1997.

Index

Abnormal sensation, 56–59, 69

Abnormal tendon reflexes, 61

Accommodating disability, 139–66;
Americans with Disabilities Act
(ADA), 149–54, 151t, 158, 159, 160,
161; Americans with Disabilities Act
Amendments Act (ADAAA), 152;
anti-ADA sentiments, 152–53, 160;
civil disobedience tactics, 149; diversity of disability rights activists, 149–
50; employment and workplace
accommodations, 158–60; examples of
steps to remove barriers, 154t; Fair
Housing Amendments Act (1988),
161; history of disability rights movement, 147, 148–49; home and family
issues, 160–64; income support programs, 135, 141, 154–57; Medicaid
program, 138, 141, 155, 157; the
onion, 141–43, 160–61; public

transportation, 157–58; Quickie
wheelchairs and the disability rights
movement, 127; Rehabilitation Act
(1973), 148–49, 152; societal attitudes
toward disabilities, 141–42, 143–48;
universal design principles, 147–48

ACTH (adrenocorticotropic hormone),
76–77

Acupuncture, 91

Acute exacerbations. *See* Flares of MS

ADA (Americans with Disabilities Act),
149–54, 151t, 158, 159, 160, 161

ADAAA (Americans with Disabilities
Act Amendments Act), 152

Adrenocorticotropic hormone (ACTH),
76–77

AFO (ankle-foot orthotic), 107–8

African Americans, 27, 30

Alternative therapies, 90–93

Alto, Joe, 139–40, 141, 150, 155, 159

About the Author

LISA I. IEZZONI, MD, is a Professor of Medicine at Harvard Medical School and Director of the Mongan Institute for Health Policy at Massachusetts General Hospital in Boston. Dr. Iezzoni has written several books, including *When Walking Fails*, and she is a member of the Institute of Medicine in the National Academy of Sciences.